High blood pressure

D1448245

Dr Vernon Coleman's
healthbooks
for all the family

HIGH BLOOD PRESSURE

by

DR VERNON COLEMAN

SEVERN HOUSE PUBLISHERS

This first world edition published 1985 by
SEVERN HOUSE PUBLISHERS LTD, of
4, Brook Street, London W1Y 1AA.

British Library Cataloguing in Publication Data

Coleman, Vernon
High blood pressure: Dr. Vernon Coleman's
medical handbooks for all the family.
1. Hypertension
I. Title
616.1′32   RC685.H8

ISBN 0-7278-2063-X Cased
ISBN 0-77278-2065-6 Pbk

To Alice and Tom and to the memory of Dick,
Harry and Timmy

Printed and bound in Great Britain by
Butler & Tanner Ltd, Frome and London.

Contents

Note

It is estimated that up to twenty per cent of the world's population have high blood pressure.
Only fifty per cent know it.
Only twenty-five per cent are being treated.
Only twelve and a half per cent are being treated effectively.

What is high blood pressure?

In order to survive and to thrive, the tissues and organs of the human body need regular supplies of fresh blood. It is blood that brings the oxygen and other essential foodstuffs without which the tissues would die, and it is blood that carries away the many waste products that are made. To travel around the body, through a complicated network of arteries, veins and capillaries, blood has to be kept under pressure. It is, of course, the heart which maintains that pressure, and it does this by regular, rhythmic pumping.

Under normal circumstances several factors affect the pressure at which blood travels around the body. First, there is the heart pump itself. If it is beating unusually rapidly or with exceptional force then that will obviously increase the pressure on the blood. Second, there is the size of the blood vessels, and in particular the muscular walled arteries. If the bore of an artery has been narrowed by muscular contraction then obviously the blood will have to be put under greater pressure for it to travel through the artery. Third, there is the amount of blood in the body. If the amount of blood increases for some reason then the pressure will rise: if the amount of fluid falls then the pressure will fall.

Under normal circumstances blood pressure varies considerably. If, for example, you are being chased by a mugger then your body, recognising that your tissues need larger amounts of oxygen to cope with the crisis, will raise your blood pressure. This temporary variation will help you to stay alive. Once you have escaped from the mugger your blood pressure will go back to normal. Such a temporary change in blood pressure is acceptable and useful. It can, quite literally, help save your life.

Unfortunately, blood pressure sometimes goes up and stays up. And that can cause all sorts of problems. The tissues and organs around the body will be subjected to excessive pressures and there is a real risk that they will be damaged. If left unchecked, a persistent rise in blood pressure can kill. It is, for example, a major cause of heart disease and of strokes. High blood pressure may not be an exciting, fashionable or dramatic disease and it may not attract much attention in the press or on television but it is one of the major causes of death in the Western world.

This book is designed to tell you everything you need to know about the causes of high blood pressure and about the available treatments. For, make no mistake about it, high blood pressure can, in almost all cases, be treated both safely and effectively. Most important of all it can, in many cases, be controlled without the use of drugs or other outside aids.

Fact-file on high blood pressure

What are the symptoms?

Most people who have raised blood pressure have absolutely no symptoms at all. That is why high blood pressure is sometimes known as the 'silent killer'.

The only symptom that is reported with any regularity is a headache, usually at the back of the head and most often said to be worst in the mornings. Apart from that (and even the significance of the headache is disputed by some physicians) the only other symptoms sometimes experienced are dizziness and tiredness.

Individuals who have had persistent high blood pressure for some time will have symptoms produced not by their high blood pressure but by a problem or disease *caused* by the raised blood pressure. So, for example, patients may develop urinary problems (having to get up at night to pass urine, or drinking a good deal) because of kidney damage, or they may develop the sort of chest pains or breathlessness suggestive of heart disease. Occasionally, patients with high blood pressure may have strokes and may develop paralysis.

It is because high blood pressure is often quite symptomless that it is particularly important for it to be detected as early as possible by screening and routine check-ups. In this way it can be dealt with before any damage is done to the body.

How blood pressure is measured

The instrument used for measuring blood pressure is called a sphygmomanometer. When having your blood pressure taken you will normally be asked to sit down or lie down and relax as much as you possibly can. (Research in Italy has shown that when a doctor in a white coat approaches a patient the patient's blood pressure will usually rise.)

Once you are properly relaxed a rubber bag in a cloth sleeve will be wrapped around your upper arm and a rubber tube from that attached to the sphygmomanometer itself. (There are mercury, aneroid and electrical machines available, by the way, but the nature of the machine does not really affect the way the reading is measured.) As air is pumped into the bag the pressure inside the rubber bag is measured.

Then, while releasing air from the bag, the person taking your blood pressure will place a stethoscope over the main artery in your arm so that he can measure the pressure under which blood is travelling around your body. Systolic pressure is the point at which he first hears blood managing to force itself through the flattened artery. The second, the diastolic pressure, is the point at which the sound fades away, eventually to disappear entirely.

There is no such thing as 'average' blood pressure since readings vary with age. It is also known that different doctors and nurses, taking the same individual's blood pressure will come up with different readings. So it is important that the same person takes your blood pressure every time.

When your doctor checks your blood pressure he may also look into your eyes. He does this because the retina at the back of the eye is covered with many small arteries. This is, indeed, the only place where the condition of the arteries can be inspected. Your doctor may also check your urine (to see if there are any signs of kidney damage) and take a chest X-ray and electrocardiograph to see if your heart has been affected by your blood pressure.

Malignant or essential

There are two main types of high blood pressure: malignant and essential.

Malignant, much the rarer of the two and also known as accelerated or secondary, is usually much the higher and more threatening of the two. There are usually signs of some damage to the body's organs. This type of high blood pressure usually develops fairly rapidly and can kill. Although it may be difficult to isolate the specific cause of malignant high blood pressure the basic problem often involves the kidneys where some physiological or pathological malfunction results in the over-production of a substance called renin. The over production of renin results in a retention of salt, a rise in the volume of blood and a constriction of blood vessel walls.

In about ninety-five per cent of cases of high blood pressure it will be of the essential type. In these cases there will be no specific identifiable cause.

It is malignant high blood pressure that usually needs hospital attention. Essential high blood pressure will usually be treated without any need for an appointment with a hospital specialist.

I must stress that both types of high blood pressure, malignant and essential, can usually be treated extremely effectively. Undiagnosed high blood pressure is a major killer. Once diagnosed it can usually be tamed.

Does high blood pressure affect life expectancy?

Your body can cope with temporary increases in blood pressure very well. A permanent increase in blood pressure can, however, cause severe damage and reduce your life expectancy.

At the age of thirty-five a man with a blood pressure of 120/80* can expect to live another forty-one and a half years. At the same age a man with a blood pressure of 150/100 can expect to live another twenty-five years.

At the age of forty-five a man with a blood pressure of 120/80 can expect to live another thirty-two years. A man of the same age with a blood pressure of 150/100 can expect to live another twenty and a half years.

At the age of fifty-five a man with a blood pressure of 120/80 can expect to live another twenty-three and a half years. A man

---

*These two figures represent the readings obtained when measuring the highest and lowest pressures at which blood is being pumped around your body. The highest figure is the 'systolic', the lowest the 'diastolic'.

of the same age with a blood pressure of 150/100 can expect to live another seventeen and a half years.

For women the figures are similar although slightly less dramatic.

At the age of forty-five a woman with a blood pressure of 120/80 can expect to live another thirty-seven years. A woman of the same age with a blood pressure of 150/100 can expect to live another twenty-eight and a half years.

At the age of fifty-five a woman with a blood pressure of 180/100 can expect to live another twenty-seven and a half years. A woman of the same age with a blood pressure of 150/100 can expect to live another twenty-three and a half years.

A lot of other factors affect life expectancy but these statistics do highlight the dangers of high blood pressure.

How high blood pressure will affect your life

Until your blood pressure is under control you should take care not to get too excited, not to expose yourself to extraordinary stresses (changing job or moving house) and not to start to take violent exercise. Any one of these circumstances will send your blood pressure up. Obviously, if your pressure is already high the additional rise could prove dangerous.

Sex is naturally one area that worries patients with high blood pressure (and, inevitably, it worries their partners too).

It is, of course, perfectly true that energetic sexual activity puts an extra strain on the circulatory system. In practice major problems during intercourse are relatively rare. But that does not mean that the risk should not be acknowledged or taken seriously.

When patients do collapse, develop heart disease or have a stroke during intercourse it is usually because the circumstances are in some way exceptional. So, for example, the older man who eats too much, drinks too much and then tries to impress a young girl with his virility will be at risk. Patients having extra-marital sex (where the feelings of guilt are greater than usual) are particularly at risk.

In general, my advice to patients with high blood pressure has to be that they should enjoy a normal, healthy sex life but

14

remember that until their blood pressure is under control they may need to be a trifle cautious and perhaps even restrained in their love making. Avoid drinking too much or eating a lot before sex and avoid adultery and sexual practices likely to lead to extra stress.

Incidentally, some drugs used to control high blood pressure may produce temporary problems – such as impotence. If this happens report to your doctor straight away.

Apart from encouraging patients to adapt their lifestyle according to the Blood Pressure Control Programme (see pages 58–82), the only other advice I would give is that they should try to get up slowly when they have been in bed or in an armchair (changing position changes the blood pressure and can produce sudden dizziness) and take warm, rather than hot, baths since immersion in very hot water can cause a sudden change in blood pressure.

What causes high blood pressure?

Only in a relatively small number of instances of high blood pressure can specific, identifiable causes be found. There may, for example, be an inherited anatomical problem offering some exceptional obstruction to the flow of blood around the body thereby affecting the overall blood pressure. The adrenal glands which have the job of producing the sort of hormones which stimulate a response to stress and danger may be diseased in some way and may, in consequence, over produce their vital hormones – with the result that the body reacts as though it were constantly under pressure. If there are too many red cells in the blood because of some internal production problem then the blood will be too thick and the blood pressure will rise accordingly because pushing thick, cell-heavy blood around the body requires extra pressure.

In the majority of cases of high blood pressure, however, no identifiable cause can be found. And although researchers are currently getting closer and closer to an understanding of just how and why the blood pressure does rise (one leading theory at the moment involves a suggestion that patients who have high blood pressure have an internal, inherited problem which prevents them from dealing effectively with calcium) we still have no real idea about how high blood pressure develops.

What we do know, however, is that in the ninety-five per cent of cases where high blood pressure develops without there being any logical physiological or pathological explanation there are very often identifiable factors which link various groups of patients together. Whether or not these factors are themselves linked in some way is still a mystery.

On the pages which follow I shall deal with the commonest and most important factors known to cause a rise in blood pressure. If you are a sufferer it is important to read through these pages carefully and see if you can spot which causes are likely to be responsible for your particular case. Once you have identified the factors which you think could be responsible for your high blood pressure you should turn to the appropriate advice. (See pages 59–79.) By changing your lifestyle in some way it will very probably be possible for you to bring your blood pressure down to normal again. A high proportion of those patients who have high blood pressure for which there is no straightforward explanation will be able to reduce it to normal simply by identifying causative factors and then dealing with those factors in the ways suggested. And even in those patients where the blood pressure cannot be controlled by dealing with causative factors it will almost always be possible to obtain some improvement by following the advice that I have listed.

Understand what is causing your high blood pressure and you stand a very good chance of being able to control it without drugs of any kind.

Genetics

No one really knows just how high blood pressure is transmitted from generation to generation but there is now little doubt that it is quite possible to inherit a tendency to develop high blood pressure. If your father or your mother had high blood pressure then you have a greater than average chance of developing it yourself.

If both your parents had high blood pressure then, it seems, your chances of developing it are even greater.

All this means that if you do not have high blood pressure yourself but you have close relatives who have high blood pressure (parents and brother and sisters) then you should have your blood pressure checked once a year as a routine precaution. Similarly, if you yourself have high blood pressure then you should encourage your own close relatives to visit their doctor once a year for a check-up.

Incidentally, according to the latest information available it seems most likely that when an individual inherits high blood pressure it is because he has inherited either a susceptibility to salt or a sensitivity to stress. So when high blood pressure runs in a family it might be sensible for all concerned to take particular note of these two factors.

What is perhaps even more remarkable – according to two experts in London – is that we probably acquire our adult blood pressure relatively early in our lives. It seems that if we are destined to end up with high blood pressure as adults we will have had a higher than average blood pressure throughout childhood. By the time we reach eighteen our future destiny is well and truly settled.

All this suggests that since high blood pressure is a major cause of death and disease in the Western world, and is now recognised to have reached epidemic proportions in many parts, we ought to be screening school children for early signs of a blood pressure problem. It would be relatively simple for children to be screened in their mid-teens and would, in financial terms, prove a sound proposition since the saving on medical manpower and materials would be massive.

Personality

During recent years, researchers all around the world have been trying to find out whether or not there is any fundamental difference between the sorts of individuals who develop peptic ulcers, the types who get cancer and the sorts who end up with high blood pressure.

It is, after all, relatively rare for one individual to suffer from more than one major disease. So it is reasonable to assume that some physical or mental characteristic must decide which particular problem will affect which individual.

The evidence which has been accumulated so far suggests that the most important factor is personality.

Psychologists and psychiatrists and trained observers of all kinds now claim that it is possible to predict just what sort of person ends up with asthma, arthritis or depression. This information is valuable for two reasons.

First, because we know now what sort of people get asthma, for example, we can pick out those individuals, and help them reduce their risks of exacerbating that particular problem. It is not possible to change anyone's personality, of course, but it is often possible to adapt or alter one's attitudes, habits and behavioural patterns. And, of course, it is also possible to reduce other risk factors. So, for example, with someone whose personality marks him as a asthma risk avoiding cigarettes is a priority.

Second, once an individual has been diagnosed as suffering from a particular ailment (such as high blood pressure) it is often possible to help that individual get better by teaching him how to adapt his approach to life. If your personality, attitude and approach to life have caused a specific problem then by altering them you can often solve or lessen it.

The following list of traits is not intended to provide a pen picture of all high blood pressure patients, of course. It is unlikely that any one patient will fit perfectly into the pattern that has been recorded (and, indeed, it is possible for an individual who has none of these personality traits to develop high blood pressure for there are, of course, factors other than personality involved).

However, if you are a sufferer look through this list and see whether or not you recognise yourself or your own behavioural pattern. Later on (See pages 59–64) I will include some advice on just how to adapt your attitudes to help reduce your blood pressure.

● People who are prone to high blood pressure, are, like people who are prone to heart disease, often quite aggressive and competitive. If you are competitive you are probably very ambitious as well. That in itself is not necessarily dangerous, of course. But if you find it difficult to relax and to stop pushing yourself to succeed then you probably do have a problem which needs dealing with.

● You may well need to do everything quickly. High blood pressure sufferers tend to be impatient and to get irritable when they are slowed down or frustrated by others. So, for example, people who get high blood pressure tend to get very irritated when they find themselves in traffic jams – and that does not do their blood pressure any good at all.

● If it is your personality that has made you liable to high blood pressure then you probably find it difficult to relax. You may even feel guilty if you sit down and do nothing. You may feel the urge to keep moving all the time and to be doing something 'useful' every minute of the day. You probably hate holidays by the sea where people lie around all day doing nothing. And you probably feel more comfortable if you have got some work with you or if you can hurry from cathedral to museum and back again.

● You are almost certainly extra sensitive to stress. For years many people have been bewildered by the fact that some individuals seem to cope extremely well with enormous amounts of stress and others crack up when the stress levels are still modest. The simple truth is, of course, that we all respond differently to stress and we all have different stress thresholds.

It is not the amount of stress we are subjected to which causes the problems, so much as our ability to cope with it. If you have a fairly low stress threshold you are likely to suffer even if your job and home life are relatively peaceful. Just missing a bus or finding that a button has come off a shirt will be enough to cause you worry and anxiety. If you have a high stress threshold you will be able to cope perfectly well with circumstances which might put someone else in hospital.

It is not particularly comforting to know this but if you are the sort of individual who suffers badly from stress and pressure then you can at least console yourself with the thought that if you ever get stranded on a desert island or stuck in the jungle you would probably survive much better than someone who does not respond to stressful situations. If you are the sort who suffers when under stress then you probably have good reflexes, you probably wake up quickly if a sudden noise breaks the stillness of the night and your body probably reacts fairly rapidly to physical danger. All those responses would make you more capable of coping in an environment where physical danger was the main threat. Unfortunately, those responses make you ill-equipped to cope with twentieth-century living.

However, do not despair. Even if you do over-react to stress there is still much that you can do to protect yourself. (See pages 64–70.)

● You probably become angry fairly easily and you may well shout when you are cross. You probably over-react sometimes and find yourself getting a little out of control. In extreme cases high blood pressure sufferers have hair-trigger tempers.

● A large percentage of the people who get high blood pressure repress their negative emotions. So, for example, when you are upset or sad you may refuse to cry, and refuse to let people see just how upset you really are. This sort of attitude is particularly prevalent among males who will almost certainly have been taught as boys to suppress emotions.

● You probably carry more guilt than is your fair share. Individuals who suffer from blood pressure problems tend to be happy to take the blame when things go wrong, they tend to worry about what other people think and they tend to be unselfish.

● You are almost certainly a worrier. You probably worry about just about anything that comes your way. You worry about whether or not you are going to have enough money (even if you have enough for your needs); you worry about the weather; you worry about whether you are doing a good job; you worry about whether other people are happy. And, of course, you worry about having high blood pressure.

Remember, of course, that not all blood pressure sufferers will exhibit all these personality traits. But look through the list and see just which ones apply to you. Then you can find out how to adapt your personality so that you can cope more effectively with life. (See pages 59–64). And do remember too, by the way, that I am not suggesting that any of the traits mentioned here are bad ones. Some of these are traits which make you a good, reliable, honest individual. These are not traits which need to be eradicated. But when problems like high blood pressure ensue they will need controlling a little.

Stress

I firmly believe that one of the most important (if not *the* most important) reasons for the apparent epidemic of high blood pressure these days is the fearful increase in the amount of stress we all have to cope with.

That may sound a strange argument. After all, most of us these days have plenty of food to eat, we have somewhere warm and dry to sleep every night and we do not have to worry too much about being attacked or eaten by wild animals. Compared to our ancestors we would, on the surface, appear to have an easy life. You would not really think that we were more likely to suffer from stress-induced diseases than our ancestors, would you?

I think the reason why we do suffer so much, and why blood pressure is now one of the commonest and most dangerous disorders in the Western world, is that our bodies were not designed for the sort of stress we have to endure these days. We were designed for an instant world.

If you turn a corner and come face to face with a man-eating tiger then your body will react remarkably well to that instant threat.

Your heart will beat faster in order to ensure that as much blood as possible reaches your muscles (this will ensure that plenty of oxygen reaches the tissues which need it to help you cope with the emergency); acid will pour into your stomach (this ensures that any food there is converted into usable energy and reaches your blood stream just as speedily as possible); and your muscles will tense (to ensure that you are well prepared for fighting the tiger, running away from it or climbing up the nearest tree).

Those are just three of the natural, physical responses your body makes to stress. There are many more.

Now, in the sort of world our ancestors lived in a few thousand years ago that sort of response would have helped to keep them alive. If you could run, fight and climb then you had a good chance of surviving. Those traits were handed down from father to son simply because the individuals who were not very good at running, jumping, climbing and fighting (in other words the individuals whose muscles did not tense and whose hearts did not beat faster) were all eaten by marauding, man-eating tigers.

Unfortunately, in our modern world those natural, automatic responses are not always appropriate. Indeed, they are sometimes a hindrance rather than a help.

The trouble is that we have changed our world far quicker than our bodies have been able to evolve. Revolutionary changes in navigation, medicine, science, military tactics, agriculture, industry and so on have changed the world a great deal. These days there are not many man-eating tigers wandering around. And most of our threats and problems cannot be solved by physical action.

The simple truth is that we have changed our world too much. Our bodies have just not been able to cope. Today we respond to danger in exactly the same way that our ancestors responded thousands of years ago. But today the dangers and threats are different.

These days we do not have to worry about being eaten: we have to worry about paying our bills, keeping our jobs, coping with inflation, fighting off court summonses, policemen and traffic wardens, and dealing with the million-and-one administrators and bureaucrats who impinge on our lives.

Our bodies respond to these modern threats in exactly the same way that they would have responded to a man-eating tiger: the heart beats faster, the blood pressure goes up, the muscles become tense and so on.

Unfortunately, these responses, although perfectly natural, are quite inappropriate.

If you have bills to pay, a job to find or a parking ticket to pay, those natural, physiological responses will not help you at all. Increased muscle tension and a higher blood pressure will help you run or fight. But those responses will not help you deal with piles of paperwork or officious administrators.

Worse still, because our modern problems tend to go on and on for long periods, the natural stress response remains switched on and our muscles stay tense and our hearts continue to beat faster for months or even years. The muscles remain tense, the heart beats faster and the blood pressure stays high for far too long – with the result that your body actually damages itself. What was intended as a protective response has become a damaging one.

Understand all this and it becomes easy to see why stress is one of the main causes of high blood pressure. It is also easy to see just why it is important for anyone who suffers from high blood pressure to learn how to cope with stress.

Is stress affecting your blood pressure?

Some people are much more susceptible to stress than others. While one individual will be able to cope perfectly well with an apparently endless series of major crises, another will be sent into a state of panic at the thought of missing a train or the sight of a button coming off a shirt. Our stress thresholds vary enormously and so it is helpful to know just how vulnerable you are to stress. If you have a high stress threshold you will be able to cope with tremendous pressures – indeed you may even enjoy being under a good deal of pressure. If, on the other hand, you have a low stress threshold then you will need to minimise your exposure to stress if you want to keep your blood pressure under control.

To benefit from the quiz which follows you must answer all the questions – and answer them accurately.

1　Do you get physical symptoms such as headaches, indigestion, vomiting or diarrhoea before important appointments or meetings?
   a　always
   b　never
   c　sometimes

2 When you are anxious or excited, does your:
   a   pulse race and your heart pound?
   b   your pulse increase a small amount?
   c   your pulse stay much the same as usual?

3 If you are concentrating hard on what you are doing and someone suddenly comes up behind you, do you:
   a   jump a mile?
   b   respond involuntarily but quickly get control of yourself?
   c   remain calm and unperturbed?

4 When you are frightened or anxious or upset, does your face:
   a   stay much the same as usual?
   b   go a little pale?
   c   go quite white?

5 When you are upset or nervous, do you:
   a   get butterflies in your stomach and sweat a good deal?
   b   get just one of those symptoms?
   c   get neither of them?

6 What is your reaction time like?
   a   below average
   b   average
   c   above average, very fast

7 Do you ever have difficulty in breathing when you are excited?
   a   often
   b   occasionally
   c   never

8 When you become angry or furious, does your face:
   a   stay the same as usual?
   b   redden a little?
   c   go bright red?

9 If you are waiting for an important phone call which does not come, do you:
  a become a nervous wreck?
  b get a bit edgy?
  c remain quite calm?

10 If, when you are lying in bed at night, you are suddenly woken by an unexpected noise, do you:
  a wake up quickly and completely?
  b take ages to wake up and realise what has happened?
  c wake up quickly but take a few seconds to realise exactly what has happened?

Now add up your score.

1 a3 b1 c2		**6** a1 b2 c3
2 a3 b2 c1		**7** a3 b2 c1
3 a3 b2 c1		**8** a1 b2 c3
4 a1 b2 c3		**9** a3 b2 c1
5 a3 b2 c1		**10** a3 b1 c2

If you scored between 20 and 30 you are the sort of individual who would survive well in a world where physical dangers posed a threat. You would stand a good chance of surviving in the jungle, for example, where your fast reactions would help you look after yourself. On the other hand, you are not, I am afraid, well suited for our modern world. And your high blood pressure is likely to have been caused or made worse by your response to stress. You will probably be able to reduce your blood pressure by learning to avoid excessive stress, and by learning to increase your capacity to cope with stressful situations.

If you scored between 13 and 19 then you are very much in the middle range, between the two extremes. You would probably still benefit from learning how to control your responses to stress.

If you scored 12 or less you would probably not last long in the jungle or in any sort of environment where physical threats are common. But you are fairly well adapted to life in the modern world. It is unlikely that your high blood pressure has been caused by your responses to stress.

Weight

According to one major study, if you are twenty per cent or more overweight your chances of developing high blood pressure are increased ten-fold. Equally important, there is evidence to show that it is by increasing the blood pressure that extra, excess weight produces heart disease.

For those who are prepared to lose excess weight the news is very encouraging. It has been shown that substantial weight reduction is at least as effective as any of the popularly pre-scribed 'first choice' anti-hypertensive drugs.

In other words, if an overweight patient with high blood pressure can lose that excess weight then the chances are that his or her blood pressure will return to normal.

Exactly why excess weight puts the blood pressure up is still something of a mystery but there are a couple of quite logical explanations available. First, it is perfectly possible that the blood pressure needs to go up for the very simple reason that there is more body to provide with fresh supplies of blood. If the pressure does not rise then the more distant parts of the body will not receive any blood. If you want to squirt water a long way out of a hose then you have to turn up the pressure. Second, it is also reasonable to assume that individuals who are overweight will have eaten too much salt (because they eat a lot of food) – and salt seems to be a common factor in exacerbating blood pressure problems in susceptible individuals.

Weight tables

The two weight tables that follow are designed to give you an idea about how overweight you are. Ideally, you should weigh less than the figure in the right hand column (that is appropriate to your height). If your weight is over this then it is time to lose weight.

Weight table
Women

Height (feet and inches)	Maximum weight (lbs)
4.10	123
4.11	125
5.0	127
5.1	129
5.2	133
5.3	136
5.4	140
5.5	143
5.6	148
5.7	152
5.8	156
5.9	160
5.10	164
5.11	167
6.0	170
6.1	173
6.2	176
6.3	180
6.4	184
6.5	187
6.6	190

Weight table
Men

Height (feet and inches)	Maximum weight (lbs)
5.0	140
5.1	141
5.2	143
5.3	145
5.4	147
5.5	150

Weight table
Men
Height *(feet and inches)* | *Maximum weight* *(lbs)*

Height (feet and inches)	Maximum weight (lbs)
5.6	154
5.7	160
5.8	166
5.9	170
5.10	175
5.11	180
6.0	184
6.1	190
6.2	196
6.3	200
6.4	205
6.5	209
6.6	212
6.7	215
6.8	220

Salt

It has been recognised for centuries that too much salt can cause damage. Even the Egyptian priests regarded it as a potential health hazard. The first scientists to argue that salt could cause harm were Ambard and Beaujard who, in 1904, published papers describing a link between salt consumption and high blood pressure. Despite this early start it was not until the 1940s that more clinical research work was published and the link between salt and hypertension firmly established. The problem then was that the recommended diet for hypertensives was, for many, simply too unpalatable. Patients who have symptom-free high blood pressure are notoriously (and understandably) reluctant to accept forms of treatment which are unpleasant. Trying to cut out all the foods that contain salt can result in a rather dull diet.

Until quite recently it was not just the difficulty of persuading people to stick to a salt-free diet that stopped doctors recommending such a solution for high blood pressure. Another problem was that, despite many research attempts, no one had managed to find out just why some people could eat lots of salt without it affecting their blood pressure while others seemed to suffer enormously if they ate modest amounts.

A year or two ago an explanation for this phenomenon was found. Those individuals whose blood pressure is adversely affected by salt are in some way genetically susceptible to it. They develop high blood pressure when they eat salt (and these days most of us living in the Western world eat too much salt – it just happens to play a fairly important part in the sort of diet we are used to) simply because they are extra sensitive to it and their bodies are unable to cope with the excesses.

If you suffer from high blood pressure then there must be a risk that excess salt will be making your blood pressure worse. Cut down your consumption of salt and your blood pressure will probably fall.

Cholesterol and fats

The arguments about cholesterol and fats seem to have been going on for ever. Part of the problem, at least, is that much of the information that has been made available about cholesterol and fats has been inspired by people with a vested interest in one particular point of view. Doctors, and others whose opinions carry weight are regularly bombarded with information paid for by those trying to sell butter, milk, cream and other, similar products.

The truth about cholesterol is that it probably is dangerous. I do not think anyone can really tell you exactly what effect eating cholesterol is likely to have on your blood pressure. But, on the other hand, there is a growing amount of reliable evidence to show that there is a link between the consumption of cholesterol and the development of heart disease. That must mean that anyone who has high blood pressure (and who, therefore, has a higher than average chance of developing heart disease) would be wise to steer clear of foods which are rich in cholesterol.

The facts about fat are much clearer. If you eat unlimited animal fats then you will run a much higher than average risk of having a heart attack. It is as simple as that.

The first link between fat intake and heart disease was noticed way back in the early 1950s. Since then much more evidence has been accumalated. At the last count over twenty major scientific and medical committees around the world were all agreed that we should eat less fat. Certainly, in America, where the consumption of milk, cream, butter and animal fats has fallen considerably the heart attack rate has also fallen. In Britain, where the consumption of milk, cream, butter and animal fats has remained fairly high the number of people having heart attacks has remained proportionally high.

As with cholesterol I do not think there is yet any clear evidence to show just what effect eating animal fats has on blood pressure. But the relationship between those three facts – high blood pressure, heart disease and fat consumption – is so well established that anyone with raised blood pressure would be foolish not to cut down consumption of animal fats.

Coffee

A number of reports have been published in recent years suggesting that coffee can cause high blood pressure. A recent trial organised by scientists from Germany and Switzerland has, however, confirmed that the effect of drinks containing caffeine (such as coffee) on the blood pressure is mild. On balance it seems unlikely that coffee can be held responsible for the development of high blood pressure, but sufferers would do well to cut down their coffee consumption.

Skin colour

Just why skin colour should affect blood pressure is still something of a mystery, but if you are black you are much more likely to suffer from high blood pressure than if you are white. And you are more likely to die from problems (such as a stroke or heart disease) caused by your blood pressure.

Attempts to come up with explanations for this have

produced a number of possible answers. It has been suggested, for example, that it is the stress of living in a hostile environment which produces the high blood pressure. Blacks, it is argued, are much more likely to have problems in achieving financial stability and they are more likely to be harassed by the police and by potential employers.

This theory is certainly substantiated by evidence which shows that when blacks migrate to urban areas where stress is greater they have a greater chance of developing hypertension.

Another quite logical explanation is that dietary factors are responsible. Many blacks live on a diet which contains much more salt, saturated fat and cholesterol than is healthy. Soul foods such as pork ribs, ham and salty fatback bacon are all particularly rich in salt and fat.

Smoking

Individuals who have high blood pressure and who smoke are often recommended to give it up as soon as they possibly can. There are sound, clinical reasons for this. Although the statistics vary, of course, from area to area and from patient to patient there is sound evidence to show that if you have high blood pressure then you have a twice as normal chance of having a heart attack. If, however, you have high blood pressure and you smoke then your chances of having a heart attack are multiplied by four. There is similar evidence which shows that if you smoke and you have high blood pressure your chances of having a stroke will be similarly increased.

Different doctors offer various explanations for these statistics. Some argue that smoking increases the blood pressure, others claim that smoking creates symptoms, such as nervousness, which in turn lead to higher blood pressure. Exactly what the mechanisms are is relatively unimportant, however. What is unarguable is that there is a relationship between smoking, high blood pressure, heart disease and strokes.

Also true, and far more encouraging, is the evidence which shows that if you manage to give up smoking then your chances of having a heart attack or a stroke will be dramatically reduced. There is, therefore, a very sound reason for people with high blood pressure to keep away from tobacco.

Noise

We are all more or less permanently surrounded by noise. The noise of cars, buses and lorries, the noise of machinery and office equipment and the noise of several million radio and television sets provides a background against which can be set the more spectacular noises of aircraft and road repairers.

All this noise undoubtedly has a harmful effect. It disturbs our ability to concentrate; it produces fatigue and bad temper and results in damaged hearing. It affects our ability to talk to each other and it increases our chances of having accidents. Because noise results in the tensing of muscles it can also produce headaches and high blood pressure. Research done in Germany with workers in a bottling plant has shown, quite conclusively, that there is a real link between noise and the development of high blood pressure. Even more important, however, the research showed that when the workers were given ear muffs those individuals whose blood pressure had risen made a remarkable recovery.

The message is, therefore, quite simple. If you spend your days working in a noisy environment then it is important that you do what you can to shield yourself from it. Providing yourself with some protection may well help reduce your blood pressure. If your blood pressure is normal then keeping unwanted noises out may help keep it that way.

Pregnancy

About one in four women suffer from a raised blood pressure at some stage during their pregnancy. The raised blood pressure may be accompanied by a swelling of the hands and legs and by the presence of measurable amounts of protein in the urine.

It is partly in order to detect a rise in blood pressure that expectant mothers are instructed to visit their doctors regularly during the months prior to delivery.

The treatment for this type of high blood pressure varies but most women are advised to learn how to relax, to spend some time resting each day and to avoid the consumption of salt. Some women may need to take special drugs to reduce their blood pressure but the drugs that are prescribed are ones that have been available for a number of years and are known to be absolutely safe for the developing baby.

Occasionally, when the blood pressure rises uncontrollably a woman may need to be taken into hospital to have her labour induced a little early. This is, however, relatively rare.

In most cases when the blood pressure has risen during pregnancy it will go back down again after the baby is delivered though it may recur during a future pregnancy.

Drugs

The drug most likely to cause an increase in blood pressure is the contraceptive pill and it seems that about one in twenty of pill takers will develop some form of high blood pressure. There is, indeed, a considerable amount of evidence now to show that women who take the contraceptive pill are liable not only to develop high blood pressure but also to suffer the disorders such as heart disease and strokes which are associated with hypertension.

Several specific factors have been isolated and shown to make the risks of high blood pressure developing more likely. So, for example, it is known that contraceptive pills which contain large amounts of oestrogen are particularly likely to produce problems, and that women who also smoke are especially at risk. The progestogen-only pill is significantly less likely to produce problems of this kind, although it is also slightly less efficient than the ordinary combined pill.

All women taking the contraceptive pill should have regular blood pressure checks done at intervals of six months. If a check-up shows that there has been a rise in the blood pressure then the obvious solution is to change to some other form of contraception. When the pill is stopped the blood pressure will usually return to normal within about three months.

Although the contraceptive pill is probably the commonest

and most widely known offender it is not the only drug likely to cause high blood pressure. There are a number of other drugs which can, in some patients, produce a noticeable and sometimes dangerous rise in pressure. Carbenoxolone, a drug sometimes used in the treatment of peptic ulcers, can produce blood pressure problems, particularly among patients who are prone to hypertension. Carbenoxolone is a drug usually given on prescription but there are a number of products available quite freely over chemists' counters which can cause changes in the blood pressure. The commonest drugs in this category are cold cures and nasal decongestants and it is important that patients who are prone to develop high blood pressure avoid these products.

Alcohol

A modest consumption of alcohol does not have any adverse effects on blood pressure. In fact, a couple of glasses of lager or wine each day may well help keep the blood pressure down. When the consumption of alcohol becomes heavier, however, then the pressure can be pushed up fairly considerably. (Since alcohol is usually rich in calories, heavy drinking invariably also means an increase in weight – and that in turn has an additional deleterious effect on the blood pressure.)

Doctors and drugs:
medical treatments for high blood pressure

The role of the general practitioner

Once you have been diagnosed as suffering from high blood pressure your general practitioner or family doctor will play an important part in your treatment. It is possible to buy equipment which will enable you to check your own blood pressure and so, theoretically, it would be possible for a sufferer to deal with his problem without any medical advice. That is not a course I recommend.

Whether or not your high blood pressure is first identified by your family doctor, you should visit him as soon as possible to tell him exactly what has been found. If your high blood pressure was discovered during a routine insurance examination or at a medical examination for a job then the doctor who performed the tests will probably write to your own doctor anyway. He certainly should do so.

When confronted with patients who have raised blood pressure, most general practitioners begin treatment with drugs straight away. Indeed, there are still many medical practitioners who firmly believe that all patients with high blood pressure will need to stay on drugs for the rest of their lives. Since most doctors get their information about diseases and drugs from drug companies, and since drug companies like selling products for years and years, it is hardly surprising that relatively few doctors are aware that blood pressure problems can be treated without drugs.

Whether or not your doctor suggests that you try reducing your blood pressure yourself there is nothing to stop you following my Blood Pressure Control Programme (see pages 58–82) and trying to 'help' the drug treatment that has been prescribed. You must, of course, tell your doctor what you plan to do. He is unlikely to object since nothing in the programme is controversial or in any way hazardous. The only real risk will be that your blood pressure may come down too much and you will feel rather light-headed and dizzy.

Once your high blood pressure has been diagnosed you should visit your doctor regularly so that he can keep a check on it. You should do this whether or not you are receiving any drug therapy and whether or not you are trying to reduce your blood pressure yourself.

To begin with I suggest that you visit the surgery once a week or once a fortnight. Obviously, however, you will need to be guided by your doctor as to when you should return to the surgery. In some instances the family doctor may want to see a patient every couple of days.

If your doctor gives you a prescription and tells you to return to the surgery in a couple of months time then I suggest you change your doctor. In order to have your blood pressure controlled effectively you will need to be seen regularly.

When your general practitioner checks your blood pressure at future visits he will be anxious to see just how well the treatments you have been trying are controlling your blood pressure. If, despite all your own efforts and despite the drugs that have been prescribed, your blood pressure has not fallen your doctor will probably prescribe a more powerful product.

Just when he will want to see you again will, of course, depend on exactly how well the blood pressure is controlled. If it is controlled well then you may eventually need only attend every three or six months. I do not think that anyone receiving treatment for high blood pressure should go for more than six months without having a check-up.

Because high blood pressure is a common problem and because it can usually be controlled quite effectively by using drugs or by changing your lifestyle, few patients with blood pressure problems are referred to a hospital specialist. If, however, the blood pressure cannot easily be controlled or is uncomfortably high then your general practitioner will resort to this.

Since high blood pressure is a potentially hazardous condition you should never have to wait more than one week for an appointment if it has been decided that a specialist's opinion is necessary.

Getting the best out of your doctor

Far too many patients come out of a doctor's surgery and *then* remember that they have forgotten to tell him something that was important, or to ask something they really needed to know.

There are many explanations for this, of course. First, most people worry about their health. That is perfectly natural. So, when they need to see a doctor they tend to be nervous and anxious. It is hardly surprising that they forget what they wanted to say. And, second, the advice that doctors give can be lengthy and involve such things as how to take tablets, when to come back to the surgery, what side effects to watch out for, and so on and so on.

I think that when you are going to see your doctor you should plan your visit carefully, and before going sit down for a few minutes and try to think of everything that you want to tell him – and everything you want to ask him. Then note it all down on a piece of paper.

You must, obviously, tell him about any symptoms you have. Tell him not just about the ones that seem important to you but of everything else you may have noticed too. Something that seems irrelevant to you may provide a vital clue.

On your first visit to the surgery tell him about any close relatives who also have high blood pressure, and be prepared to answer questions about your weight, your diet, your smoking habits and your daily exercise ration. If you have a past history of any disease then tell him about that too. Your doctor may have forgotten or the information may be 'lost' in your files. Your doctor will probably want to know something about your job because how you spend your day will have some effect on your blood pressure – so be prepared for questions about your work.

It is also wise to tell him about any pills, tablets or medicines you are already taking; whether they are products that have been prescribed or products that you have bought over the chemist's counter.

Remember too to jot down any specific questions that you want to ask. You may want to know whether you can carry on mountaineering, or whether you should temporarily retire from Grand Prix motor racing.

Write down all the questions you want answered. Obviously, if you go in to see your doctor clutching a huge three hundred page account of your medical history and you have hundreds of questions to ask then he is going to become a little impatient. But he will not mind at all if you go in with a few notes jotted down. Indeed, he will almost certainly appreciate the fact that you are trying to help him help you get better.

And write down the advice he gives you. If he tells you about your pills make a note of what he tells you. Make a note about the dosage, about any possible side effects, about when to stop taking the pills, about whether or not you need to avoid any particular food or alcohol while on the drugs.

Make a careful note too about when you have got to go back to the surgery, about whether or not you need to see anyone at the hospital and, if you do need to see a specialist, the name of the doctor he is referring you to.

Doctors write down everything you tell them. And there is absolutely no reason at all why you should not write down everything the doctor tells you.

Reading your prescription

Unless your doctor dispenses his own drugs you will usually be given a prescription. You will be expected to take that prescription along to a pharmacy where your drugs will be made up.

On that prescription will be written all the instructions that the chemist needs.

The name of the drug will be there, of course, together with instructions about when the drug is to be taken, whether it is to be taken with meals or before them, and so on.

Normally, those instructions would be written on the label of the bottle you are given. But, occasionally, some instructions are omitted. And that can lead to confusion.

To avoid that risk I have here included a list of the Latin abbreviations used by doctors when writing prescriptions – together with their meanings.

Now, you can read your own prescription for your blood pressure pills.

Abbreviation	Latin	English
aa	ana	of each
ac	ante cibum	before meals
ad lib	ad libitum	freely
alt die	alt diebus	alternate days
alt noct	alt noctibus	alternate nights
aqua calida	aqua calida	hot water
bal	balneum	bath
bd	bis in die	twice a day
bid	bis in die	twice a day
c	cum	with
cc	cum	with
cm	cras mane	tomorrow morning
cn	cras nocte	tomorrow night
dol urg	dolore urgente	when the pain is bad
eq	equalis	equal
f	fiat	let it be made
flav	flavus	yellow
fs	semi	half
ft	fiat	let it be made
hn	hac nocte	tonight
hor decub	hora decubitus	at bedtime
hs	hora somni	at bedtime
m	misce	mix
md	more dicto	as directed

Abbreviation	Latin	English
mdu	*more dicto utendus*	to be used as directed
mit	*mitte*	send
om	*omni mane*	every morning
on	*omni nocte*	every evening
prn	*pro re nata*	when needed
qd	*quater in die*	four times a day
qh	*quatis horis*	four hourly
qid	*quater in die*	four times a day
qq	*quaque*	every
qqh	*quarta quaque hora*	every fourth hour
qs	*quantum sufficiat*	as much as suffices
r	*recipe*	take thou
rep	*repetatur*	let it be repeated
rep dos	*repetatur dosis*	let the dose be repeated
si dol urg	*si dol urgeat*	if the pain is severe
sig	*signetur*	let it be labelled
sig	*signa*	label
sos	*si opus sit*	if necessary
ss	*semi*	half
stat	*statim*	immediately
td	*ter in die*	three times a day
tds	*ter die sumendum*	three times a day
tert qq hora	*tertia quaque hora*	every third hour
tid	*ter in die*	three times a day
ut dict	*ut dictum*	as directed

The role of the hospital specialist

Unless your blood pressure is unusually high or difficult to control you are unlikely to need to see a hospital specialist. Under some circumstances, however, you may have to.

So, for example, if your general practitioner cannot control your blood pressure with the drugs he is familiar with he may arrange an appointment with a specialist so that he can obtain some advice about other drugs to try. New products are coming onto the market every month and no general practitioner can possibly hope to keep up to date with all the latest products. Referring a patient to a hospital specialist for treatment advice is a sign of strength not weakness.

You are likely to need to go into hospital for treatment of high blood pressure under three separate sets of circumstances:

● If your doctor or your specialist suspect that there may be an underlying cause for your high blood pressure then they will probably take you into hospital for tests to be done. Some of the equipment used these days is extremely sophisticated and needs expert technicians if useful results are going to be obtained. You are also likely to need to go into hospital if your doctor finds that there is a cause for your high blood pressure and that the cause needs treatment (for example, a deformed artery that needs a surgical operation).

● If your blood pressure is unusually high then your doctor may decide that it will be better to treat your blood pressure in hospital simply so that it will be possible to bring it under control more speedily. In hospital doctors can change your treatment hourly if they wish. They can also give treatments by injection instead of by mouth and most drugs work faster when passed straight into the tissues.

● If your blood pressure is difficult to control you may need to go into hospital for a few days while different drugs are tried.

Always remember, however, that even if your blood pressure is high or difficult to control there will nearly always be a drug available which will control it. Once your blood pressure problem has been identified treatment is usually a matter of trial and error until a suitable therapeutic agent is found.

When does high blood pressure need treating with drugs?

If you asked this question of a hundred doctors you would probably receive a hundred different answers.

At one extreme there are many doctors who claim that a high proportion of patients with 'higher-than-average' blood pressure can be controlled by losing weight and reducing their exposure to stress. This is, indeed, a point of view favoured by the World Health Organisation.

At the other extreme there are those doctors (sometimes sponsored by drug companies) who believe that every patient with high blood pressure should receive drug treatment.

The World Health Organisation recommendations, which are entirely free of commercial pressure, are that patients who have a diastolic pressure below 90mm of mercury do not need treatment. Those patients who have a diastolic pressure between 90mm of mercury and 95mm of mercury need to have their blood pressure checked every three months but they do not need drug therapy.

Those patients should, of course, be given advice about diet and stress control.

Patients who have a diastolic pressure above 95 mm of mercury should, says the World Health Organisation, be started on drug treatment.

When patients do have mild to moderately raised blood pressure and are left without drug therapy the evidence that is available suggests that their blood pressure will eventually fall back to within normal levels – particularly, of course, if they have done what they can to ease their stress, improve their diet and adjust their weight.

The evidence suggests that if you have high blood pressure and your doctor prescribes for you then you should, perhaps, ask whether or not your prescription is really necessary. You should also ensure that your blood pressure is checked regularly so that as soon as it falls your treatment can be stopped or at least adjusted.

How to find out what sort of drugs you are taking

The name of the drug that has been prescribed for you should be on the bottle or box which contains your supplies. It will also have been on any prescription written out for you. First of all look through the list of generic names on pages 47–50 to see if the product you are taking is listed there. Then, if that fails, turn to pages 83–93 where most of the available branded products for the treatment of high blood pressure are listed. In this section you will see that the generic constituents of each product have been listed.

Drugs for high blood pressure

There are scores of drugs available for the treatment of high blood pressure and to be perfectly honest I doubt if there are many doctors in practice who have ever even heard of all the available products. Many patients with high blood pressure need to keep taking drugs for months or even years – that means that there are huge potential profits to be won by companies which can market safe and effective drugs. It is hardly surprising, therefore, that most of the major international companies produce at least one drug designed for the treatment of high blood pressure.

At first sight the many different products which are on the market seem very different from one another. In fact, most of the drugs available for the treatment of high blood pressure tend to fall into a small number of basic categories. These are the available groups:

DIURETICS

If your doctor can get rid of salt and fluid from your body then your blood pressure will probably fall. Diuretics are drugs designed to do exactly this – they encourage your body to excrete fluid and salt. If you take a diuretic you will usually notice that you are passing more urine than usual – for this reason diuretics are usually taken in the morning. (There is not much point in taking a drug at night if it is going to make you want to get up and urinate.)

There are a number of different types of diuretic available and they work in slightly different ways and at varying rates.

BETA BLOCKERS

The drugs in this group are now probably the ones most commonly used for the treatment of high blood pressure. Beta blockers have an effect on the heart, interrupting the passage of nerve impulses which control the heart rate. They usually tend to slow down the heart rate. Just how they affect blood pressure is still uncertain but it is fairly logical to assume that if you slow the pump the pressure will fall. One of the commonest problems with drugs for the treatment of high blood pressure is that they produce hypotension (see page 56) when patients stand up; beta blockers tend to produce a reduction in blood pressure which does not vary much whether the patient stands or lies down.

VASODILATORS

Drugs in this group work by making the arteries enlarge. Naturally, when the arteries get bigger the blood pressure must fall. (If you are pumping water through a hose and the hose suddenly widens the pressure will be bound to fall.)

Unfortunately, the body tends to try and combat this change by increasing the force at which the pump (the heart) sends blood through the arteries. Vasodilators tend, therefore, to increase the heart rate.

DRUGS ACTING ON THE NERVOUS SYSTEM ('NERVE BLOCKERS')

There are many drugs available which work by stopping nervous impulses travelling from the brain to the artery walls. Some of these drugs act on the brain itself, others work on the nerves which carry the messages directly to the blood vessels. The general effect of these products is to prevent the artery walls being contracted – and to leave them relaxed and wide, thus reducing blood pressure.

SEDATIVES AND TRANQUILLISERS

Because it is widely accepted that high blood pressure is often produced by stress and tension, doctors sometimes prescribe tranquillisers and sedatives. The benzodiazepines are probably the group of drugs most commonly used in this way (of these the best known is probably diazepam, a drug produced by many different manufacturers but still best known as Valium).

A full list of sedatives and tranquillisers would take up a disproportionate amount of space in this book but if your doctor prescribes a drug that does not appear on any of the lists then there is a good chance that it could be a tranquilliser or sedative.

These products should be used only for short periods of time. Many are addictive. Stress is much better dealt with by the techniques outlined on pages 64–70.

CALCIUM ANTAGONISTS

Some researchers now believe that patients with high blood pressure have an excess of calcium in some of their cells. A major study in Belgium recently showed that there is a correlation between serum calcium and high blood pressure.

There are now, therefore, drugs available which work by controlling calcium. (The calcium produces high blood pressure, by the way, by causing the muscle in the artery walls to contract, thereby making the vessels narrower.)

ACE INHIBITORS

These are another new group of drugs. They work by stopping blood vessels from being constricted and by reducing the volume of fluid in the vessels. They get their name from the fact that they are 'Angiotensin Converting Enzyme inhibitors'.

DRUGS WHICH AFFECT THE BRAIN (CENTRAL EFFECT)

The problem with drugs that work centrally is that they do tend to cause other, unwanted side effects. Many of the products in this category cause drowsiness, depression, a dry mouth, nasal stuffiness, impotence and a reduction in libido. These drugs are used less and less these days.

Drugs for high blood pressure: Generic list

ACEBUTOLOL: A beta blocker

AMILORIDE: A diuretic

ATENOLOL: A beta blocker

BENDROFLUAZIDE: A diuretic

BENZTHIAZIDE: A diuretic

BETHANIDINE: A 'nerve blocker'

CAPTOPRIL: ACE inhibitor

CHLORTHALIDONE: A diuretic

CLONIDINE: A central effect. In June 1984 the Drug and Therapeutics Bulletin reported that 'clonidine should not be used for the treatment of hypertension and patients already on it should be changed to alternative treatment'. One reason for this claim is that if clonidine is stopped suddenly patients can suffer dangerous side effects – the drug should, therefore, be reduced slowly and under medical supervision.

CLOPAMIDE: A diuretic

CYCLOPENTHAZIDE: A diuretic

DEBRISOQUINE: A nerve blocker

DESERPIDINE: A central effect

DIAZOXIDE: A vasodilator. Diazoxide can interfere with insulin metabolism. It is normally only used in the treatment of hypertensive emergencies.

FRUSEMIDE: A diuretic

GAUNETHIDINE: A 'nerve blocker'

HYDRALAZINE: A vasodilator

HYDROCHLOROTHIAZIDE: A diuretic

HYDROFLUMETHIAZIDE: A diuretic

INDAPAMIDE: A diuretic, and possibly also a calcium antagonist

INDORAMIN: A 'nerve blocker'

LABETOLOL: A beta blocker and 'nerve blocker'

METHOSERPIDINE: A central effect

METHYCYCLOTHIAZIDE: A diuretic

METHYLDOPA: A central effect

METOPROLOL: A beta blocker

MINOXIDIL: A vasodilator

NADOLOL: A beta blocker

NIFEDIPINE: A calcium antagonist

OXPRENOLOL: A beta blocker

PARGYLINE: This product is rather unusual in that it is a mono-amine oxidase inhibitor and these drugs are usually reserved for patients with depression. Patients taking mono-amine oxidase inhibitors need to avoid certain foods – otherwise potentially fatal interactions can occur. Patients given this drug should be given a list of those foods that they must avoid.

PENBUTALOL: A beta blocker

PHENOBARBITONE: A sedative

PINDOLOL: A beta blocker

POTASSIUM CHLORIDE: Potassium (used to replace potassium lost by some diuretics.)

PRAZOSIN: A vasodilator

PROPRANOLOL: A beta blocker

RAUWOLFIA: A central effect

RESERPINE: A central effect

SOTALOL: A beta blocker

SPIRONOLACTONE: A diuretic

THEOBROMINE: A sedative

TIMILOL: A beta blocker

VERAPAMIL: A calcium antagonist

VERATRUM: A central effect

Getting the best out of prescribed drugs

Drugs can be dangerous, it is true. But they can be extraordinarily useful. And, if drugs help bring your blood pressure down to normal then they can save your life. To get the best out of drugs, while at the same time minimising the risks you run, you need to know how to use drugs safely and effectively. Read through the following notes.

● Always make sure that you find out as much as you can about the drugs you have been given. If your doctor does not tell you when your drugs need to be taken then ask him for the information – he may forget to put the advice on your prescription. The most important things you need to know are:

1   For how long the drug needs to be taken. Usually, drugs given for high blood pressure need to be taken continuously, at least until your blood pressure is taken again and your need for the drug can be reassessed.

2   How many times a day the drug should be taken. If a drug needs to be taken once a day it is important that it is taken at the same time each day. If a drug has to be taken twice a day then it should be taken at intervals of twelve hours. A drug that needs to be taken three times a day should be taken at eight hourly intervals (unless you are instructed otherwise) and a drug that needs taking four times a day should be taken at six hourly intervals. Modern drugs are powerful and sophisticated; they need to be taken at exactly the right time if the right effects are to be obtained.

3   Whether the drug should be taken before meals, during meals or after meals. Some drugs may cause stomach problems if taken on an empty stomach – they will

obviously be safer if taken with food. Other drugs are not properly absorbed if taken with food.

● When you have been given instructions about how to take a drug follow those instructions carefully.

● Remember that many drugs do not mix well with alcohol. It is always safer to assume that you should not drink while taking a drug until you have checked with your doctor.

● You must not take non-prescribed medicines while taking prescribed medicines. The effect of some drugs for the treatment of high blood pressure can be distorted by over-the-counter remedies. Even cold cures can cause severe interactions.

● Occasionally, drugs do not mix with food. If your doctor tells you not to eat a particular type of food then it is important that you follow his instructions.

● Keep drugs in a locked cupboard where the temperature is stable. Blood pressure drugs, if taken by children, can be extremely dangerous. Although most of us keep our medicines in the bathroom that is not the best place for them – the temperature and humidity levels there tend to vary too much. Your bedroom is probably best.

● Do not remove drugs from their proper containers except when you are taking them or when you are transferring them to a special 'day' box to carry around with you.

● Some drugs prescribed for high blood pressure can cause drowsiness. If you have to drive a motor car or handle any machinery then it is important that you ask your doctor if the drugs he has prescribed you will have this side effect.

● Never, ever take drugs that have been prescribed for someone else. Even if they seem to have the same symptoms as you, even if they have a high blood pressure problem, their pills may not suit you.

● It is important that once you start receiving treatment you always try to see the same doctor. One reason for this is that if several doctors are prescribing for you the chances are that your drug regime will become complicated and confusing. Different doctors prefer different drugs for the treatment of high blood pressure. The other important reason for sticking to one doctor is that different doctors measure blood pressure in slightly different ways. If one doctor is a little deafer than another, for example, he may hear the appropriate sounds a few seconds later – and record a different reading. Also, sphygmomanometers can vary.

● Be on the look out for side effects and do remember that if you seem to develop a second illness then the chances are high that it is caused by the treatment you are receiving.

● Remember, that although drugs need to be used with care and caution they may help save your life. If you need drugs to bring your blood pressure down to normal levels then you must keep taking your drugs. The risks associated with the drugs you are taking are unlikely to be as high as the risks that you would run if your blood pressure was allowed to remain high and uncontrolled.

Side effects

A recent survey published in the British Medical Journal showed that at least forty per cent of the people who take prescribed drugs suffer some form of side effect. Most of these side effects appeared within the first four days of treatment. Some were minor and short-lasting; others were permanent, debilitating and dangerous.

The side effects suffered by patients taking drugs for the treatment of high blood pressure will obviously vary according to the individual patient and the nature of the drug prescribed. Patients should always be aware of the possibility of side effects developing and should be prepared to report new signs or symptoms to their doctors straight away. (Remember, that if side effects do occur it is always wiser to speak to your doctor before stopping treatment. It is sometimes wiser to continue with treatment and put up with the side effects than it is to stop treatment suddenly.)

Although all drugs can cause a whole range of side effects, there are some side effects which are particularly common with drugs used to control high blood pressure and these are the ones that are dealt with here.

Drowsiness
Commonest with those drugs which have a central effect

Dry mouth
Commonest with those drugs which have a central effect

Impotence
Commonest with those drugs which have a central effect and with beta-blockers

Loss of interest in sex
Commonest with those drugs which have a central effect

Loss of potassium
Commonest with some diuretics. To prevent this condition developing some doctors will, when prescribing diuretics, also prescribe potassium supplements.

Tiredness
Commonest with those drugs which have a central effect

Hallucinations
Commonest with the beta-blockers

Confusion
Commonest with the beta-blockers and some drugs having a central effect.

Hypotension
Can occur with all blood pressure drugs but least common with beta-blockers (see also page 56).

Breathlessness
Commonest with beta-blockers

If you suffer regularly from one particular type of side effect then your doctor may be able to solve the problem by switching to another type of drug.

Combination drugs

Occasionally, it is easier to control high blood pressure with a combination of two or more drugs rather than with just one. (The separate drugs will sometimes increase each other's effect.)

To make it easier for patients who need to take two separate sets of pills, many drug companies now make combination treatments which consist of two or more chemical ingredients packed together in the same tablet.

The dangers of mixing drugs

If you are prescribed a drug you should never take any other drug unless it has been prescribed for you by a doctor who knows what you are already taking.

Blood pressure drugs tend to be rather sensitive to other chemicals and mixing drugs can be dangerous. High blood pressure drugs are particularly likely to cause problems when taken together with:

> oral contraceptives
> diuretic drugs
> drugs for the treatment of diabetes
> cough medicines
> nasal decongestants
> alcohol
> drugs for the treatment of heart disease
> drugs for the treatment of depression

If you need to take a drug in one of these categories and you also need something for high blood pressure then your doctor will have to take special care to ensure that no problems result.

Drugs during pregnancy and breast feeding

If you are pregnant or planning to become pregnant or if you are breast feeding a baby you must tell your doctor. Some of the drugs used to control high blood pressure could damage your baby.

There are, however, some drugs available which can be used safely during pregnancy.

Making drug taking easier

If you need to take more than three tablets a day or if you need to break any of your tablets in half then you should ask your doctor if there are any possible alternatives. The more tablets you have to take the more likely you are to forget a dose – and the less effective your treatment will be. If you have to spend time breaking tablets into halves or quarters then your dosages will become rather irregular as it is difficult to break tablets into equal portions.

There are so many different blood pressure control drugs available on the market that your doctor will probably be able to find a product which will help you avoid spending the day swallowing pills or dissecting them on the kitchen table.

Taking drugs on time

It is important that drugs prescribed for the control of high blood pressure are taken on time.

If your doctor has prescribed drugs that need to be taken just once a day then remembering your pills should not be too difficult. If, however, he has given you drugs that need to be taken three times a day, or has given you two or more different types of pills and told you to take one lot twice a day and another lot four times a day then you may have problems.

You can help yourself keep track of your pill taking by making a small daily pill chart. The chart that follows is designed for a patient told to take tablet 1, three times a day; tablet 2, once a day and tablet 3, twice a day.

A fresh chart could be made out for each new day and the individual pills ticked off as they are taken.

	8.00am	4.00pm	8.00pm	Midnight
Tablet 1	1	1	—	1
Tablet 2	1	—	—	—
Tablet 3	1	—	1	—

Going abroad

If you are going out of the country then do remember to take a supply of your pills with you. Some of the products used to control blood pressure are not available internationally and you may find difficulty in obtaining the pills that you have found most effective.

Do remember, too, to keep your pills with you and not to leave them in your luggage. Your blood pressure will not be helped if you end up in Tahiti while your pills are sitting locked in a luggage hold in Hong Kong.

And remember, also, that in hot climates your need for blood pressure pills may be reduced. If you are planning to go somewhere hot you should tell your doctor who may, for example, be able to give you lower dose pills. Alternatively, he can tell you how to reduce your usual medication.

The hazard of hypotension

Occasionally, drugs used to bring down the blood pressure work a little too efficiently – and they reduce the blood pressure too much, producing a condition known as *hypotension*.

Patients with hypotension usually notice that they feel dizzy or light-headed. These symptoms are worse on sudden movement, as when rising out of a chair or getting up out of bed in the morning. The dizziness usually wears off after a few seconds.

The problem of hypotension is more likely to occur during the hotter weather. Then the body tries to lose heat by pushing as much blood as possible into the blood vessels of the skin. Heat is then lost from the blood and the body manages to keep its internal temperature stable. When the peripheral blood vessels are dilated the existing blood pressure must fall.

If you suffer from dizziness you should visit your doctor as soon as possible so that he can check your blood pressure and, if necessary, adjust your medication. If your hypotension only occurs when it is hot then it may simply be enough to reduce your pills during those spells.

Is high blood pressure a permanent problem?

Patients with high blood pressure always used to be told that they would need to stay on drugs for ever. I have spoken to a number of patients over the years who have been threatened with all sorts of horrible consequences if they ever dared consider coming off their tablets. 'If you stop taking your pills you will have a stroke,' is a common enough comment from doctors brought up to believe that the only way to deal with high blood pressure is by taking pills.

The truth is very different.

Although we still do not really know what causes high blood pressure in a strictly scientific sense (we do not know what sort of physiological process is involved) we do know that there are a number of specific factors which are often responsible for the development of high blood pressure. (Some of the commonest factors are listed on pages 15–34).

And we also know that if these factors are controlled then the blood pressure can often be reduced to normal levels again. With the result that it will be possible to stop taking drugs.

So high blood pressure need not be a permanent problem. Nor do I think that patients with high blood pressure need resign themselves either to taking drugs for the rest of their lives or else dying early from a stroke or a heart attack.

Having said that, do not stop taking your drugs if you have been prescribed them. Before trying to reduce your own blood pressure to safer levels you must first ask your doctor's advice. While changing your lifestyle have your blood pressure checked regularly so that your medication can be adjusted. If and when your blood pressure pills need to be reduced then they must be reduced by your doctor and he must do so while keeping a close eye on your blood pressure.

Blood Pressure Control Programme

Introduction

There is much that you can do to help yourself if you suffer from high blood pressure. There is a very real chance that if you follow the advice in this Blood Pressure Control Programme you will be able to control your blood pressure without drugs.

Before starting this programme you must, of course, consult your doctor. As your blood pressure is reduced your need for drugs may change.

Adapt your personality

Earlier (see pages 17–21), I explained how your personality can affect your chances of developing high blood pressure. There are many other factors which decide whether or not you are going to develop high blood pressure but 'personality' is undoubtedly a critical one. And even though I do not pretend for an instant that you can *change* your personality (nor do I think that it would be a good idea to try) you can certainly *adapt* it and your way of life in such a way that your blood pressure will benefit.

AGGRESSION AND COMPETITIVENESS

In order to cope with your ambitions you must first decide what your priorities are; and decide which parts of your life are most important. If you let your ambitions spill over into every aspect of your life then you will soon burn yourself out. So, for example, if your job is extremely important to you it is important that you are able to relax when you are playing games. If you take everything seriously you will be pushing yourself too hard – and your blood pressure will rise.

And remember too that however important your ambitions are you will be much more likely to succeed if you are prepared to take time off occasionally to relax. Read the sections which deal with physical and mental forms of relaxation. (See pages 64 and 69). If you are an aggressive, ambitious individual then it is important that you read these parts of the book carefully. In addition to spending some time each day relaxing you would probably be wise to put time aside for more complete relaxation. So, for example, make sure that you have a half day every week when you do something that really does not matter too much. And when you are planning to go on holiday try not to get carried away and give yourself too many things to do.

Finally, do learn to recognise the signs which tell you that you are pushing yourself too hard. There may not be any symptoms to show just what is happening to your blood pressure but look out for other symptoms that show that you are making too many demands of your mind and body.

Look, for example, for signs such as indigestion, headaches, nausea, sleeplessness, and tiredness. Those can all be signs that you are putting yourself under too much pressure. If you can get one it might be wise to buy a machine to measure your own blood pressure. (See page 81.) You will then be able to see what happens to your blood pressure under different circumstances. That should give you a good idea of just what you can manage without damaging your health.

FRUSTRATION

Many of the problems that produce frustration can be avoided by a little advance planning. When you are organising something complicated (such as a house move or a dinner party) make a list of all the things that have to be done. And then go through your list carefully, looking for possible areas where things can go wrong. Then try to ensure that you have prepared contingency plans for dealing with these potential problems.

Do not allow yourself to become too dependent on others, either. These days we all have to be dependent on many other people – and strikes or failures of supplies can easily lead to frustration. If a power dispute is starting then make sure that you have alternative forms of heating and lighting around. If your business depends on one particular product try to make sure that you have an alternative supplier available.

If you have an important appointment to keep make plans to travel early and do something else in the time that may (all being well) be spent waiting.

None of this advice means changing your personality, of

course. All it involves is adapting the way you live to ensure that you suffer as little frustration as possible. That is bound to have a beneficial effect on your blood pressure.

DIFFICULTY IN RELAXING

This is one of the commonest problems of all. Part of the problem is that many of us think of relaxation as being something rather 'odd'. But to relax, you do not have to do anything strange; you do not have to wrap your legs around your ears and you do not have to join any strange religious organisation. All you have to do is read the advice on pages 64–69.

STRESS

If you think you are particularly sensitive to stress (and you can find out just how sensitive you are by doing the quiz on page 23) then read the instructions on pages 64–70.

TEMPER

If you are the sort of individual who gets easily aroused then you should probably learn to get rid of your aggressions in as harmless a way as possible. It is not sensible to try to repress your natural aggressions but neither is it particularly sensible to let your aggression out when you are working or socialising – you are likely to annoy people, make enemies and store up extra stresses and strains for yourself.

There are plenty of harmless ways by which you can rid yourself of your aggressive feelings. Take up an active sport, for example, and get rid of your aggressions by slamming a squash ball around or by hammering a tennis ball to death. Or buy a supply of old plates and keep them in the garage or in a shed down the garden; then, next time you are feeling angry, smash plates until you feel better. Or take up gardening and go and do a little heavy digging when you feel like shouting. Or buy yourself a punch-bag, paint a face on it and pummel that the next time you want to shout or scream at someone. (Some factories and offices have 'angry' rooms these days where workers can get rid of their aggressions.)

Do remember, however, that if you suffer from high blood pressure you should not do anything too physically exhausting!

REPRESSED EMOTIONS

Do not store up tears inside you. There is now evidence to show that when we cry there are very good reasons for it: not only does our crying make it clear to those around us that we need extra comfort and attention but the tears we shed contain harmful substances that our body needs to get rid of when we are upset. The research work in this area is still in its infancy but it does seem possible that if you refuse to cry your body will store up harmful chemicals and you will end up with a genuine, full blown depression.

I am not suggesting that you open the floodgates at every possible opportunity. But do not be afraid to cry in front of those who are close to you, or in private. Store up the tears and you will probably make your blood pressure go up.

GUILT

First of all you must, of course, decide whether or not any particular feeling of guilt is really justified or not. Obviously, if you are feeling guilty because of something that you have done (run into a parked car or broken a cup, for example) then the only solution is to apologise and make what amends you can. In most instances, however, guilt is far more complex than that. If you are the sort of individual who tends to suffer from guilt then you probably feel guilty because of things you have not done and because of your own suspicions about how other people will feel and respond.

This is the type of guilt that causes most pain and to deal with it you must first of all find out exactly why it is you feel guilty. Is it because you feel that you have failed someone such as your mother, your employer, your spouse or your God? Much of the guilt we suffer is produced by our relationships with those who are very close to us (love is the greatest single cause of guilt) and so in order to protect yourself more effectively you must learn to differentiate between the realistic expectations of those who are close to you and their unrealistic demands. You must learn not to allow other people to put unreasonable demands on you or your conscience.

So, for example, you should perhaps not feel guilty if you cannot visit your parents every week, if you cannot buy your children all the toys they want, if you cannot do all the overtime that your employer would like you to do – and so on.

The truth about individuals who suffer a lot from guilt is that they tend to be thoughtful and caring people.

If you suffer a lot from pangs of guilt it is probably because you care too much about other people; you probably worry too much about what other people want; about what other people feel and about how your actions are going to be seen by others.

I know that this may sound strange, but to protect yourself a little and to keep your blood pressure under control you need to be a little more selfish, a little more self-aware and a little more able to appreciate your own good points. If you are the sort of individual who is driven by guilt then you are probably conscientious, hard working, ambitious, thoughtful, reliable, honest and generous. Despite all these good points you probably think of yourself as a failure and you are probably far too critical about what you do. You probably expect far more from yourself than you would ever dream of expecting from anyone else – and some of the people around you may well take advantage of this trait.

I suggest that you sit yourself down and write out a list of your good points. Pretend that you are writing your own obituary and be honest and fair to yourself. You will almost certainly end up with a fairly long list of good things that you could say about yourself. Now, being equally honest and impartial, try to list all your bad points.

Next time you are swamped with guilt look at your list, take a little pride in yourself and learn to be a little more selfish. Your blood pressure will benefit enormously.

WORRY AND ANXIETY

Fears can be debilitating – and have a bad effect on your blood pressure. To cope with your fears you must recognise and face those things that worry you most. The unknown, unidentified fear is much more dangerous and more damaging than the fear that has been carefully examined.

Once you have made a list of all the things that really worry you, you can go through that list and see what you can do to help yourself worry less. So, for example, if you worry a good deal about your health it might be wise to visit your doctor for a complete check up. Or, better still, make a positive decision to learn more about your body and to come to terms with just what you need to do in order to conquer your problems. Self awareness and understanding will last much longer in your battle against fear than professional reassurance.

If your fears concern money, employment or whatever, the same is true. Once you have made a precise list of all the things that worry you then you are more likely to be able to do something to help yourself. You will not be able to solve all your fears or eradicate all your worries straight away, of course. But you will be able to do something to help yourself. And that always makes a tremendous difference to the way your body and your blood pressure respond.

Learn to relax your body

Stress, muscle tension and high blood pressure are all closely interlinked. If you learn how to relax your muscles then you cannot only get rid of some of your anxiety but you may also be able to reduce your blood pressure.

To relax your muscles you must first learn just how your muscles feel when they are tight and tense. To start with, clench your fist. As you do you will feel the muscles of your hand and forearm tighten and become firm. Now, gradually let your fist unfold. This time you will feel the muscles slowly relax. To relax your muscles, all you have to do is to stiffen and then relax them group by group.

When you first start relaxing you should choose a quiet, private place where you are not likely to be interrupted and where stimuli are least disturbing. It is difficult to relax in a crowded department store or on a busy train – although you will probably be able to do that eventually.

Start by lying down in a darkened room where you are likely to be left alone for at least a quarter of an hour – you should allow a quarter of an hour for each session to start with and you will need to plan on spending that much time every day for a week or so until you have mastered the art of physical relaxation.

Here is the step-by-step programme for physical relaxation.

1 Clench your left hand as firmly as you can, making a fist with your fingers. Clench it hard and you will see your knuckles turning white. Then gradually let your fist unfold and as you do so you will feel the muscles relax.

2 Bend your left arm so that your biceps muscle stands out. Then relax and let the muscles ease. Let your arm lie loosely by your side and try to ignore it.

3 Relax your right hand in exactly the same way.

4 Relax your right biceps muscle in the same way.

5 Tighten the muscles in your left foot. Curl your toes. When the foot feels as tense as you can make it, let it relax.

6 Tense the muscles of your left calf. If you reach down you can feel the muscles at the back of your leg firm up as you tense them. Bend your foot back at the ankle to help tighten up the muscles. Then let the muscles relax.

7 Straighten your leg and push your foot away from you. You will feel the muscles on the front of your thigh tighten up; they should be firm right up to the top of your leg. Then let the muscles relax.

8 Tense and relax your right foot.

9 Tense and relax your right lower leg.

10 Tense and relax your right thigh.

11 Lift yourself up by tightening up your buttock muscles. You will be able to lift your body upwards by an inch or so. Then let the muscles fall loose again.

12 Tense and contract your abdominal muscles. Try to pull your abdominal wall as far in as possible. Then let go and allow your waist to reach its maximum circumference.

13 Tighten the muscles of your chest. Take a big, deep breath and strain to hold it for as long as possible. Then let go.

14 Push your shoulders back as far as they will go, then turn them forwards and inwards. Finally, shrug them as high as you can. Keep your head perfectly still and try to touch your ears with your shoulders. It will probably be impossible but try it anyway. Then let your shoulders relax and ease.

15 Next, tighten up the muscles of your back. Try to make yourself as tall as you possibly can. Then let the muscles relax.

16 The muscles of your neck are next. Lift your head forward and pull at the muscles at the back of your neck. Turn your head first one way and then the other way. Push your head back with as much force as you can. Then let the muscles of your neck relax. Move it about to make sure that it really is loose and easy.

17 Move your eyebrows upwards and then pull them down as far as they will go. Do this several times, making sure that you can feel the muscles tightening both when you move the eyebrows up and when you can pull them down again. Then let them relax.

18 Screw up your eyes as tightly as you can. Pretend that someone is trying to force your eyes open. Keep them shut tightly. Then, keeping your eyelids closed, let them relax.

19 Move your lower jaw around. Grit your teeth. Wrinkle your nose. Smile as wide as you can, showing as many teeth as you have got. Now let all those facial muscles relax.

20 Push your tongue out as far as it will go; push it firmly against the bottom of your mouth and the top of your mouth and then let it lie relaxed and easy inside your mouth.

As you do all these simple exercises remember that your breathing should be slow, deep and regular.

You will probably begin to feel calmer and more relaxed after just one session of physical relaxation. But remember that you really need to persist with this physical relaxation programme. As you become more experienced you will not have to relax step-by-step but will be able to relax your whole body more or less instantly.

Learn to relax your mind

One of the easiest and most effective ways to deal with stress and to stop anxiety, fear and worry affecting your blood pressure is to learn how to relax your mind. There is now evidence from all parts of the world to show that patients with high blood pressure have learned to control their pressure simply by learning how to relax their minds – many, many patients have been able to stop taking drugs simply by using mind relaxing techniques.

Under normal, everyday circumstances an unending stream

of facts and feelings pours into your mind. Even when you are not consciously 'thinking', your eyes, ears, nose and other sense organs will be pushing thousands of bits and pieces of unwanted information into your mind. Together, all these pieces of information help to produce stress and pressure. If you can cut out the number of messages going into your brain then you will be able to ease the amount of pressure on your mind. And the effect on your blood pressure will almost certainly be beneficial.

Many of the people who recommend mental relaxation suggest that you should try to empty your mind completely in order to cut out the damaging effect of all this information.

The problem is, of course, that trying to empty your mind of all the conscious and subconscious messages that keep streaming into it is not easy. Indeed, very many people find the prospect of emptying their minds completely so terrifying that they never even try. And so they lose the possibility of benefiting from simple mental relaxation.

Fortunately, however, there is another way to cut down the amount of damaging information pouring into your mind. And that is to fill your mind with pleasant, peaceful, relaxing thoughts. In other words, all you have to do is re-learn how to daydream. I say 're-learn' deliberately because you will almost certainly have been able to daydream when you were small. But you were probably taught (by both your parents and your teachers) that daydreaming is wasteful and rather naughty.

Daydreaming works for several reasons. First, it works because your body will respond to an imagined world just as effectively as it will respond to the real world. When the film *Lawrence of Arabia* was shown in the cinemas a few years ago, cinema managers around the world were astonished to find that the sales of cold drinks and ice creams rocketed. Even when the heating failed in one particular cinema and the temperature plummeted the patrons still wanted to buy cold drinks and ice creams. The explanation was that the cinema patrons were responding to the desert scenes that they were watching on the screen. Their bodies responded as though the desert was entirely real. So, fill your mind with some pleasant, relaxing, imaginary scene and your body will respond as though the scene were real. The horrors of the real world around you will be forgotten.

The second reason why daydreaming works so well is that the human body responds positively to good, happy, feelings. When we are frightened or worried we respond badly: our blood pressure goes up, we feel upset, we get indigestion and so on. But when we are happy and contented there is a very clear and useful healing effect on the body. So, if you learn how to daydream you will benefit in both those ways.

And your blood pressure will very probably come down.

When you begin re-learning how to daydream you will probably have to find yourself somewhere quiet and peaceful. You will need to be able to cut out the world. Later on, when you have mastered the art, you will be able to do it just about anywhere.

So, to start with, lie yourself down on your bed, close the door, take the telephone off the hook, feed the animals and draw the curtains. Put a 'Do Not Disturb' notice on the door.

Once you are peacefully settled try to remember some particularly happy and peaceful scene from your past. It is best to use a real scene because you will be better able to re-create all the necessary feelings. But you can, if you like, use an entirely fictional scene.

If you are using a scene from your past then you might try a beach scene from a good holiday by the sea. With your eyes firmly closed take big, deep breaths as slowly and as regularly as you possibly can. And then slowly try to feel the warmth of the sun on your face. Try not to let anyone else into your daydream by the way. If you let people into your daydream then you are likely to either end up with a nightmare or with a fantasy. And neither is likely to be particularly relaxing.

Once you can feel the sun on your face try to imagine that you can hear the sound of the waves breaking on the shore. And try too to feel the warm, soft sand underneath you. Listen to the seagulls circling overhead and smell the salty sea air. Allow a gentle breeze to play over your body.

Once your mind has been convinced your body will be convinced too. The accumulated pressures from the real world will slowly disappear. As your mind is filled with all these peaceful thoughts so your body will begin to respond. Your blood pressure will begin to fall.

You do not, of course, have to restrict yourself to this one particular daydream. You can build up your very own, personal library of useful daydreams. There can be real memories, there can be fictional memories and there can be memories taken from films or books. It does not matter what the memory is as long as the effect is to make you feel happy and peaceful, and as long as you can create memories that are convincing.

Reduce your stress by organising your life

The motorist who remembers to buy petrol for his car and put air into the tyres will be far less likely to find himself stressed by running out of fuel or having a 'blow-out' on the motorway. The shopper who knows in advance what he is going to buy will be far less likely to end up making a second trip to the shops. The businessman who plans ahead will be far less likely to end up with a 'crisis' on his hands. Bad organisation and poor planning often lead to anxiety, to increased stress loads and to high blood pressure. Learn to organise your life and you will reduce the number of crises which might make your blood pressure go up.

Follow this simple four-stage plan.

1 Keep a diary that contains details of all events that need advance planning (birthdays, anniversaries etc). Get into the habit of examining it each morning to make sure that you know just what you have to do. Advance planning for trips and meetings of all kinds obviously helps to reduce the risk of something going wrong.

2 Keep an efficient filing system to enable you to store bills, letters and receipts just where you can find them. There is nothing more frustrating (and worse for your blood pressure) than hunting around for an important letter and wasting hours on the job. You do not have to buy a filing cabinet – you can use old brown envelopes or a cardboard box.

3   When you have a really difficult problem to solve do not let it ruin your life – simply write down all the possible solutions in a notebook. Keep the list somewhere safe and near to you and add new solutions as they occur to you. Keep the list by you when you are in the bath, in the car or in bed: those are the places where ideas tend to come to you. Then, when you finally need to make a decision take a look down your list of possibilities and you will probably find that one particular answer stands out. You will certainly be able to cross out many of the alternatives which seemed logical when you wrote them down but which by now look silly.

4   Keep a notebook and a pencil with you at all times. Jot down any thought that needs remembering or needs action. When they are put down on paper, problems always seem slightly less significant. And you will not have to worry about remembering them either.

Control your weight

Losing weight can make a dramatic difference to blood pressure. Indeed, it is one of the most effective ways to reduce it.

There are two ways of losing excess weight.

The first is to increase the amount of work and exercise that you do while keeping your food intake fairly stable. You need to increase your daily exercise regime fairly substantially, however, in order to burn up food faster than you are taking it into your body. This is, I know, the solution that many people favour these days and a large number of the joggers who set out each morning in their track suits and woolly hats hope to lose weight. Unfortunately, exercising is not a practical or particularly effective way of losing weight. The sad truth is that to lose weight by exercising you have virtually to become a professional athlete, forever running, lifting and working out. A little, occasional, mild exercise just will not make any real difference.

The second solution is to reduce your food intake so that it falls below your body's requirements. Do this and your body will need to take food from your stored supplies – and you will lose weight.

The problem with this sensible, sound and efficient solution is, of course, that eating less than you need can be difficult and even painful.

Before I explain how I think you can manage to lose weight relatively painlessly and easily I want to go on and discuss the other major problem that all dieters have to face – keeping the food intake down afterwards so that the excess weight does not come back straight away. Losing weight is, like giving up smoking, very easy: hundreds of thousands of people do it many times a year. The difficult part is *staying* slim. The reason why I want to discuss this problem now is that if you understand why you are likely to put weight back on again after dieting then you will not only understand the sort of things which make your dieting fail but you will also understand what you need to do to lose weight without too much pain or discomfort.

Anyone wanting to lose weight should know that there is an appetite control centre in the human brain which is designed to ensure that you eat exactly what your body needs and in precisely the quantities that are needed. Research done in America showed quite conclusively that when children are allowed to eat exactly what they want and in the quantities they want they neither put on excess weight nor do they acquire any of the many, common digestive troubles which seem to plague us all these days.

Children will, it is perfectly true, eat a diet that looks unbalanced. One day they will eat nothing but ice cream. Another day they will eat nothing but apples. And so on. But over a period of some months the diet they eat is perfectly balanced. Indeed, one research project has shown that a child's natural eating habits matched the sort of diet that dieticians would choose if they had the chance.

Other research has shown that this appetite control centre is so sophisticated that it can change your diet if your circumstances change. So, for example, research done with soldiers has shown that when men are suddenly put down in the desert or in the Arctic wastes they will unconsciously change their dietary habits to fit in with their circumstances. Their bodies' needs vary according to the environment and the appetite control centre makes the appropriate signals to adjust dietary habits.

The reason why so many of us get fat is that we eat the wrong foods, at the wrong times and in the wrong amounts. And we do this because we eat for all the wrong reasons. We eat food that looks good; we eat foods that have been promoted on television; we eat up everything on our plates whether or not we are hungry simply because when we were small we were told by our mothers that we should never leave food to go to waste; we eat at fixed meal times that are often decided by other people; we eat because other people are eating and we want to look sociable; we eat because we are upset and we have always associated food with feeling good and so on and so on.

In other words we no longer listen to our appetite control centres; we eat for all the wrong reasons.

And this explains not only why so many of us are overweight, but why we so often find it difficult to keep weight off once we have dieted successfully. As soon as we have finished dieting we simply go back to our old, bad habits and we put all the weight back on again.

If you are going to lose your excess weight and keep it off then you have to get back into the habit of eating according to your body's needs and not eating according to other people's wishes. You have to learn to listen to your body's internal signs of hunger, learn to break bad eating habits, and learn to eat the foods you need, when you need them and in the quantities you need.

To maintain your weight you need to follow these rules:

1   You must concentrate on what you are doing when you are eating. If you are reading, talking or watching television while you are eating you will miss the all-important messages from your appetite control centre.

2   You must make absolutely sure that you only ever eat when you are hungry. Every time a piece of food is on its way to your mouth you must ask yourself whether or not you are

genuinely hungry. If you are hungry – then eat it. If you are not really hungry but you are eating for some other reason then stop.

3   Never, ever be frightened to leave food on the side of your plate if you have had more than you need. I know it is a waste to throw food away but its just as much a waste (and likely to do your body untold damage) to eat it. This is something that most of us find difficult to do – largely because we were taught as children that it is sinful to waste food. Fortunately, when you find that you are having to leave food on the side of your plate you can easily solve the problem for the future by serving yourself smaller portions.

4   You are better off eating small meals regularly than huge meals every now and then. If you eat occasionally your body will store up excess food because it will know that it might be some time before more food comes its way. If you eat small meals fairly regularly the food will be burnt up quite quickly. Nibbling is better for you than stuffing yourself at meal times.

5   Do make sure that you never use food as a crutch. Do not promise yourself food as a prize or a reward. Do not eat to cheer yourself up. It is an easy habit to form but a difficult one to break.

Following these simple instructions will take a little effort to start with. If you have spent years of your life acquiring bad eating habits it will take longer to get into the habit of eating sensibly.

The reward, though, is that your weight will remain stable. And, hopefully, your blood pressure will remain under control.

If you want to lose weight then you have somehow to trick your appetite control centre into thinking that you have put enough food into your body. You must convince yourself that you are no longer hungry, even though you have eaten less food than your body needs. If you can do this then your body will draw on stored fat supplies and you will lose weight.

There are several simple tricks that you can try.

When you feel hungry eat filling but low-calorie snacks.

Drink a glass of one-calorie squash or cola; or a cup of black coffee or lemon tea; or a bowl of clear soup. You will feel full without having filled your body with calories.

Another trick is to have a small snack half an hour before a main meal. A piece of chocolate or raw fruit, or a hunk of vegetable will do. The aim is to spoil your appetite, convince your body that you are no longer hungry and stop you eating as much as you really need.

You can also help yourself by picking foods that take a lot of chewing (foods such as raw vegetables). This will slow you down and make you more aware of when you have eaten enough.

Reduce your salt intake

The evidence now available suggests that anyone who has high blood pressure should make an attempt to reduce his salt intake. This is best done by avoiding the following foods (or, at least, keeping their consumption down to a minimum):

> processed foods in general
> canned foods
> junk foods (such as take away hamburgers etc)
> crisps
> salted peanuts
> cheese crackers
> chips
> lobsters
> oysters
> salted butter and cheese
> sausages
> bacon
> milk and milk products

You should also avoid adding salt when cooking food. And salt should be banished from the table.

If you find saltless food unappetising there are a number of other flavourings that you can try. These include:

> lemon juice
> parsley
> garlic

74

horseradish
tarragon

Increase your potassium intake

Just as there is evidence to show that too much salt has an adverse effect on patients with high blood pressure so there is also evidence to show that some patients with blood pressure problems are deficient in potassium. Increase your consumption of foods that are rich in potassium. These include:

apples
apricots
asparagus
avocados
bananas
beans
brussels sprouts
cabbage
corn on the cob
dates
grapefruit
oranges
peas
peppers
prunes
potatoes (though not as fatty, salted chips!)
radishes
raisins

Reduce your intake of cholesterol

You can cut down your intake of cholesterol in two ways.

First, by cutting down the consumption of foods which are themselves rich in cholesterol. This means avoiding foods on the following list as much as possible:

cheese
chocolate
eggs
cream

shellfish
caviare
brains
hearts
kidneys
liver
sweetbreads

You do not have to cut out your consumption of these foods completely – but you do need to cut down.

Second, by drastically cutting down your consumption of animal fats such as butter, milk, cooking fat, dripping and lard. These fats are all converted into cholesterol in your body.

Reduce your intake of animal fats

Do not listen to those cleverly thought out messages telling you to 'drink a pint of milk a day' or to eat cream cakes because although they are 'naughty' they are 'nice'.

Animal fats can kill and you need to keep your intake of such products to a minimum. You should eat less:

fatty meat
eggs
butter
milk
cream
margarine (except ones containing polyunsaturated fats)

You should also grill rather than fry your food when possible. And you should cook with vegetable oils.

While you are cutting down on these foods increase your consumption of chicken, fish, fruit and vegetables.

Reduce your caffeine intake

Caffeine shrinks blood vessels and has an adverse effect on blood pressure levels. I do not think there is any need to cut out caffeine completely but if you are drinking more than three or four cups of strong coffee or tea each day or you drink many cola drinks then you should try to cut down.

Control your intake of alcohol

You should not drink more than two or three glasses of alcohol (beer, wine, spirits) in any one day. If you drink less than this on one day do not transfer that 'allocation' to another day.

Stop smoking

Any method you choose that works is a good one! Some people claim that they have managed to give up smoking by visiting a hypnotist; others that special chewing gum helped them more than anything else. I once came across a man who managed by eating prunes. Heaven knows what sort of effect that had on his bowels but it apparently helped him 'kick' the tobacco habit.

Before you try to give up find out exactly why you smoke. If you do it to help you relieve your stress then giving it up without doing anything else to help you cope with stress will simply result in a likely increase in your blood pressure – rather than a decrease. If you usually inhale when you are smoking then you are very probably addicted to tobacco, and, for you, giving up smoking is likely to be a physical strain. If you rarely smoke by yourself but merely smoke when you are with friends then your habit is probably a social one.

Once you have decided just why you smoke – and you have done what you can to ensure that giving up smoking is not likely to have a damaging effect on your life – then you can set up the practical business of giving up tobacco.

The techniques described below are ones that have been found to work, but, as I say, any method that works is a good one.

1 If you have an economical mind then you will probably find that it helps to write down each day just how much money you have saved (or would have saved) by not smoking. It adds up quickly and by the end of a month the amount will be substantial.

2   If you usually smoke one particular type of cigarette try changing the brand you buy every time you buy a new pack. This will make life rather difficult because you will be constantly looking for new brands. It will also make smoking a less familiar occupation. Some cigarettes will be weaker: others stronger. Buy them from a different shop, too. Never buy more than one pack at once; buy in packs of ten; and try to remember to forget to take your cigarettes with you when you go out.

3   Make a list of all the places where you smoke. Put every single place on your list – bedroom, car, restaurant, office, bus, train, lavatory, lifts, streets, shops, friends homes, bathroom, garden, pub, telephone kiosks etc. Then write out the places again, this time with the places where you do least smoking at the bottom, and the places where you do most at the top.

Now, stop smoking in each place in turn, starting with the one that is at the bottom. So, for example, if it is the garden make sure that you do not smoke there on day one. Put a tick by 'garden' to remind you just how far you have got. Then, on day two, do not smoke in the place that is next to the bottom. If, for example it is the bathroom make sure that you do not smoke there.

And carry on, day by day, working your way up the list. You must remember, of course, that as you go up the list you cannot smoke anywhere that you have already ticked. So, on day three, for example, you cannot smoke in the garden or the bathroom or in the place that is third up the list.

The main advantage with this system is that it will enable you to give up at an acceptable rate. Even if you do not manage to give up smoking altogether you will have managed to give up a bit – and that will help. The other advantage is that it allows you to carry on smoking in those places where you *need* to smoke most of all. So, if your office is right at the top of your list and that is where you are under most stress and most likely to need the comfort of a cigarette you will be able to smoke there right until the end.

Remember, too, as you give up smoking that even if you can only cut down (rather than give up altogether) that will have a noticeable effect on your health and will reduce the risk of your blood pressure giving you major problems in the future.

Take up gentle exercise

A good deal of nonsense has been talked about exercise in recent years. Everywhere you turn there are actresses, singers and minor celebrities insisting that they have a secret exercise solution to good health. The leotard business has never been better and there are hundreds of pushy entrepreneurs selling rowing machines, weight lifting contraptions, track suits, running shoes and all sorts of other gadgets.

The claims that have been made by all these 'experts' have made exercise sound like a universal panacea. Whether they are encouraging you to take up aerobic exercise, gymnastics, weight lifting or squash, the experts will insist that their sport will help you live longer, stay fitter and avoid problems like high blood pressure.

I am afraid that a good deal of this talk has been based not on sound clinical and scientific principles but on commercially inspired rhetoric. The truth is that jogging and running are so bad for the majority of us that track suits should have Government health warnings stitched onto them. I could show you a pile of cuttings an inch thick to support *that* contention. I would like to see those advocating violent exercise as a cure for all ills produce a tenth as much evidence in support of their arguments.

There are two main problems with the sort of exercise that is recommended by the exercise enthusiasts. First, they invariably seem to insist that it is vital to go through the pain barrier in order to benefit from an exercise programme. I contend that it is positively dangerous to try and go through a real pain barrier and that people who insist on following this sort of foolhardy advice will end up injuring themselves. Pain is one of the body's natural defence mechanisms. When we exercise and we get a pain the pain is there for a purpose – it is designed to make us stop what we are doing.

The exercise freaks argue that if you continue to exercise you can force your way through the pain barrier.

I agree with them on this point but the fact is that when anyone goes through the pain barrier the body produces its own pain relieving hormones simply because it is under the impression that a major crisis requires the body to keep moving. If a soldier hurts his ankle while running across a battle field his first reaction will be to stop and rest his ankle for a while. If, however, he is being chased by enemy soldiers he will want to get up and carry on running. His body, recognising that the need to keep running over-rides the need to protect the damaged ankle, will produce internal pain relieving hormones. The pain of the injured ankle will be temporarily forgotten.

This is why marathon runners can keep going when they have injured themselves. The problem is, of course, that by continuing to run on the injured joint the runner is damaging the joint. He may end up with a serious injury that will require long-term, professional treatment. (The injured soldier running away to save his life would probably damage his joint too but he would probably be quite happy to accept such a small price in return for his life.) This is why approximately one third of all joggers and runners need specialist orthopaedic or osteopathic treatment every year.

The second reason why the exercise enthusiasts often do more harm than good is that they invariably take themselves far too seriously. Many of the people who take up exercise to get fit become quite dedicated to their sport. They become anxious to do well and they put themselves under stress to run faster, lift more weights, or beat another player at tennis, badminton or squash.

Anyone who has high blood pressure will probably be under enough stress from other areas in their life without adding more from this source.

Having said that, gentle, regular exercise, taken for fun and enjoyed as a form of relaxation, will help anyone suffering from high blood pressure.

There is not, I am afraid, any evidence to show that exercise actually helps reduce blood pressure. But many sufferers have found that gentle exercise does give them a feeling of well being and there are certainly many doctors happy to recommend it.

Just what sort of exercise you choose should depend on your personal preferences. Cycling, swimming and dancing are three quite excellent, natural types of exercise that many people enjoy. If you are not sure what to try then I suggest walking. Do not set yourself targets or push yourself if you think you have had enough, and do remember that if walking reduces your blood pressure then you may feel a little dizzy and need to rest occasionally. Remember, when you start your modest exercise programme, that if you enjoy your exercise it will undoubtedly reduce your stress levels. So you will benefit twice!

Keep a check on your own blood pressure

Measuring your own blood pressure at home has several advantages:

1 You can take weekly readings which will give you a more accurate picture of your blood pressure than readings taken once every three or six months at a doctor's surgery.

2 Most people's blood pressure rises automatically when they go into a doctor's surgery. Taking your blood pressure at home enables you to avoid this problem.

3 If you take your own blood pressure and keep a chart of your readings you can see how effective your Blood Pressure Control Programme is.

4 You will save time and so will your doctor.

5 If you become skilled at measuring your own blood pressure you should be able to check the blood pressure of your relatives.

6 You can make sure that you always take your blood pressure at the same time of day. (Blood pressures vary from one time of day to another. It tends to be highest at about ten am and lowest at about three am.)

Several types of sphygomanometer are available for home use. Check yours alongside your doctor's machine.

Wear a medical bracelet or necklace

I suggest that patients who are regularly treated with drugs wear some form of identification bracelet, carrying details of their condition and of treatment they are receiving. Some pharmacies sell suitable jewellery. Otherwise ask your doctor for details of the Medic Alert Foundation. This organisation sells bracelets upon which can be engraved a brief summary of your condition together with the telephone number of the Foundation. In an emergency doctors can telephone the Foundation for more detailed advice and information about your condition.

Alternative treatments

I know of no safe and efficient 'over the counter' drugs for the treatment of high blood pressure. Its treatment is one area where orthodox medicine really does have the best – and only – answers.

Alternative or complementary forms of medicine are playing an increasingly large part in medical care but there are no, that I know of, alternative forms of treatment which match the types of treatment offered by orthodox medical practitioners.

Appendix

Drugs for the treatment of high blood pressure

The following list consists of the brand names of products prescribed for the treatment of high blood pressure. Under each brand name I have listed the constituent drugs and the manufacturers. (See also pages 45-56.)

If you need further information about a drug and your doctor is unable to provide you with it then I suggest that you write to the Medical Director of the company concerned.

ABICOL
Pink tablets
They contain: *reserpine and bendrofluazide*
Manufacturer: Boots Company PLC, Thane Rd, Nottingham NG2 3AA

ADALAT RETARD
Pink tablets
They contain: *nifedipine*
Manufacturer: Bayer UK Ltd, Strawberry Hill, Newbury, Berks RG13 1JA

ALDOMET
Yellow tablets
They contain: *methyldopa*
Manufacturer: Merck Sharp and Dohme Ltd, Hertford Rd, Hoddesdon, Herts EN11 9BU

ANGILOL
Pink tablets
They contain: *propranolol*
Manufacturer: DDSA Pharmaceuticals Ltd, 310 Old Brompton Rd, London SW5 9JQ

APRESOLINE
Pink tablets and yellow tablets
They contain: *hydralazine*
Manufacturer: Ciba Laboratories, Horsham, West Sussex
RH12 4AB

APSOLOL
Pink tablets
They contain: *propranolol*
Manufacturer: APS Ltd, Whitcliffe House, Whitcliffe Rd,
Cleckheaton, West Yorkshire BD19 3BZ

APSOLOX
White, yellow and orange tablets available
They contain: *oxprenolol*
Manufacturer: APS (see above)

BARATOL
Blue tablets and green tablets
They contain: *indoramin*
Manufacturer: Wyeth Laboratories, Huntercombe Lane South,
Maidenhead, Berks SL6 OPH

BEDRANOL
Pink tablets
They contain: *propranolol*
Manufacturer: Lagap Pharmaceuticals Ltd, Old Portsmouth
Rd, Peasmarsh, Guildford, Surrey GU3 1LZ

BERKOLOL
Pink tablets
They contain: propranolol
Manufacturer: Berk Pharmaceuticals Ltd, St Leonards Rd,
Eastbourne, East Sussex BN21 3YG

BETA-CARDONE
Green, red or white tablets available
They contain: *sotalol*
Manufacturer: Duncan, Flockhart and Co Ltd, 700 Oldfield
Lane North, Greenford, Middlesex UB6 OHD

BETALOC-SA
White tablets
They contain: *metoprolol*
Manufacturer: Astra Pharmaceuticals Ltd, Home Park Estate, 'King's Langley, Herts WD4 8DH

BETIM
White tablets
They contain: *timolol*
Manufacturer: Edwin Burgess Ltd, Leo Laboratories Ltd, Longwick Rd, Princes Risborough, Bucks HP17 9RR

BLOCADREN
Blue tablets
They contain: *timolol*
Manufacturer: Merck, Sharp and Dohme Ltd (see above)

CAPOTEN
Mottled white tablets
They contain: *captopril*
Manufacturer: E.R. Squibb and Sons Ltd, Squibb House, 141-149 Staines Rd, Hounslow TW3 3JB

CATAPRES
White tablets
They contain: *clonidine*
Manufacturer: Boehringer Ingelheim Ltd, Southern Industrial Estate, Bracknell, Berks RG12 4YS

CO-BETALOC
White tablets
They contain: *metoprolol* and *hydrochlorthiazide*
Manufacturer: Astra Pharmaceuticals Ltd (see above)

CORDILOX 160
Yellow tablets
They contain: *verapamil*
Manufacturer: Abbott Laboratories Ltd, Queenborough, Kent ME11 5EL

CORGARD
Pale blue tablets
They contain: *nadolol*
Manufacturer: E.R. Squibb and Sons Ltd (see above)

CORGARETIC 40
Mottled white tablets
They contain: *nadolol* and *bendrofluazide*
Manufacturer: E.R. Squibb and Sons Ltd (see above)

DECASERPYL
White or pink tablets
They contain: *methoserpidine*
Manufacturer: Roussel Laboratories Ltd, Wembley Park, Middlesex HA9 ONF

DECASERPYL PLUS
White tablets
They contain: *methoserpidine* and *benzothiazide*
Manufacturer: Roussel Laboratories Ltd (see above)

DECLINAX
White or blue tablets
They contain: *debrisoquine*
Manufacturer: Roche Products Ltd, PO Box 8, Welwyn
Garden City, Herts AL7 3AY

DOPAMET
Yellow tablets
They contain: *methyldopa*
Manufacturer: Berk Pharmaceuticals Ltd (see above)

ESBATAL
Peach coloured tablets
They contain: *bethanidine*
Manufacturer: Calmic, Crewe Hall, Crewe, Cheshire CW1
1UB

HARMONYL
Pink tablets
They contain: *deserpidine*
Manufacturer: Abbott Laboratories Ltd (see above)

HYDROMET
Pink tablets
They contain: *methyldopa, hydrochlorothiazide*
Manufacturer: Merck, Sharp and Dohme Ltd (see above)

HYPOVASE
White or orange tablets
They contain: *prazosin*
Manufacturer: Pfizer Ltd, Sandwich, Kent CT13 9NJ

INDERAL LA
Lavender and pink capsule
They contain: *propranolol*
Manufacturer: ICI Pharmaceuticals PLC, Alderley Park, Macclesfield, Cheshire SK10 4TF

HALF-INDERAL LA
Lavender and pink capsules
They contain: *propranolol*
Manufacturer: ICI Pharmaceuticals PLC (see above)

INDERAL TABLET
Pink tablets
They contain: *propranolol*
Manufacturer: ICI Pharmaceuticals PLC (see above)

INDERETIC
White capsules
They contain: *propranolol* and *bendrofluazide*
Manufacturer: ICI Pharmaceuticals PLC (see above)

INDEREX
Pink and grey capsule
They contain: *propranolol* and *bendrofluazide*
Manufacturer: ICI Pharmaceuticals PLC (see above)

ISMELIN
White or pink tablets
They contain: *guanethidine*
Manufacturer: Ciba Laboratories (see above)

LASIPRESSIN
White tablets
They contain: *frusemide* and *penbutolol*
Manufacturer: Hoechst UK Ltd, Salisbury Rd, Hounslow, Middlesex TW4 6JH

LONITEN
White tablets
They contain: *minoxidil*
Manufacturer: Upjohn Ltd, Fleming Way, Crawley, Sussex RH10 2NJ

LOPRESOR
Pink or blue tablets
They contain: *metoprolol*
Manufacturer: Geigy Pharmaceuticals, Horsham, West Sussex RH12 4AB

LOPRESOR SR
Yellow tablet
They contain: *metoprolol*
Manufacturer: Geigy Pharmaceuticals (see above)

LOPRESORETIC
White tablets
They contain: *metoprolol* and *chlorthalidone*
Manufacturer: Geigy Pharmaceuticals (see above)

MEDOMET
Yellow tablets
They contain: *methyldopa*
Manufacturer: DDSA Pharmaceuticals Ltd (see above)

MODUCREN
Blue tablets
They contain: *hydrochlorothiazide, amiloride,* and *timolol*
Manufacturer: Thomas Morson Pharmaceuticals, Hertford Rd,
Hoddesdon, Herts EN11 9BU

NATRILIX
Pink tablets
They contain: *indapamide*
Manufacturer: Servier Laboratories Ltd, Windmill Rd,
Fulmer, Slough SL3 6HH

PRESTIM
White tablets
They contain: *timolol* and *bendrofluazide*
Manufacturer: Leo Laboratories Ltd (see above)

RAUTRAX
Red tablets
They contain: *rauwolfia, hydroflumethiazide, potassium chloride*
Manufacturer: E.R.Squibb and Sons Ltd (see above)

RAUWILOID
Buff tablets
They contain: *rauwolfia*
Manufacturer: Riker Laboratories, Morley St, Loughborough,
Leics LE11 1EP

RAUWILOID & VERILOID
Red brown tablet
They contain: *rauwolfia* and *veratrum*
Manufacturer: Riker Laboratories (see above)

SECADREX
White tablets
They contain: *acebutolol* and *hydrochlorothiazide*
Manufacturer: May and Baker Ltd, Rainham Rd South, Dagenham, Essex RM10 7XS

SECTRAL
White tablets
They contain: *acebutolol*
Manufacturer: May and Baker (see above)

SECTRAL CAPSULES
Buff and white capsule or buff and pink capsule
They contain: *acebutolol*
Manufacturer: May and Baker (see above)

SECURON
Yellow tablets
They contain: *verapamil*
Manufacturer: Knoll Ltd, The Brow, Burgess Hill, Sussex RH15 9NE

SEOMINAL
Yellow tablets
They contain: *phenobarbitone, theobromine* and *reserpine*
Manufacturer: Winthrop Laboratories, Sterling Winthrop House, Onslow St, Guildford, Surrey GU1 4YS

SERPASIL
Blue tablets
They contain: *reserpine*
Manufacturer: Ciba Laboratories (see above)

SERPASIL ESIDREX
White tablets
They contain: *reserpine* and *hydrochlorothiazide*
Manufacturer: Ciba Laboratories (see above)

SLOW PREN
White tablets
They contain: *oxprenolol*
Manufacturer: HN Norton and Co Ltd, Patman House, George Lane, South Woodford, London E18 2LS

SLOW TRASICOR
White tablets
They contain: *oxprenolol*
Manufacturer: Ciba Laboratories (see above)

SOTACOR
Blue tablets
They contain: *sotalol*
Manufacturer: Bristol-Meyers Pharmaceuticals, Station Rd, Langley, Slough, Berks, SL3 6EB

SOTAZIDE
Blue tablets
They contain: *sotalol* and *hydrochlorothiazide*
Manufacturer: Bristol-Meyers Pharmaceuticals (see above)

SPIROPROP
Pink tablets
They contain: *propranolol* and *spironolactone*
Manufacturer: Searle Pharmaceuticals, Lane End Rd, High Wycombe, Bucks HP12 4HL

TENORET 50
Brown tablets
They contain: *atenolol* and *chlorthalidone*
Manufacturer: Stuart Pharmaceuticals Ltd, Carr House, Carrs Rd, Cheadle, Cheshire SK8 2EG

TENORETIC
Brown tablets
They contain: *atenolol* and *chlorthalidone*
Manufacturer: Stuart Pharmaceuticals (see above)

TENORMIN
Orange tablets
They contain: *atenolol*
Manufacturer: Stuart Pharmaceuticals (see above)

THIAVER
Blue tablets
They contain: *veratrum* and *epithiazide*
Manufacturer: Riker Laboratories (see above)

TOLERZIDE
Lilac tablets
They contain: *sotalol* and *hydrochlorothiazide*
Manufacturer: Bristol Meyers Pharmaceuticals (see above)

TRANDATE
Orange tablets
They contain: *labetalol*
Manufacturer: Duncan, Flockhart and Co Ltd (see above)

TRASICOR
White, yellow or orange tablets
They contain: *oxprenolol*
Manufacturer: Ciba Laboratories (see above)

TRASIDREX
Red tablet
They contain: *oxprenolol* and *cyclopenthiazide*
Manufacturer: Ciba Laboratories (see above)

VERILOID
Yellow tablets
They contain: *veratrum*
Manufacturer: Riker Laboratories (see above)

VISKALDIX
White tablets
They contain: *pindolol* and *clopamide*
Manufacturer: Sandoz Pharmaceuticals, 98 The Centre, Feltham, Middlesex TW13 4EP

VISKEN
White tablets
They contain: *pindolol*
Manufacturer: Sandoz Pharmaceuticals (see above)

Index